Industrial Housewives:
Women's Social Work
in the Factories
of Nazi Germany

The *Women & History* series:

- *Beautiful Merchandise: Prostitution in China 1860-1936*, by Sue Gronewold

- *The Empire of the Mother: American Writing about Domesticity 1830-1860*, by Mary P. Ryan

- *Women, Family, and Community in Colonial America: Two Perspectives*, by Alison Duncan Hirsch and Linda Speth, with an Introduction by Carol Berkin

- *Votes and More for Women: Suffrage and After in Connecticut*, by Carole Nichols, with a Foreword by Lois Banner

- *A New Song: Celibate Women in the First Three Christian Centuries*, by JoAnn McNamara

- Dames Employées: *The Feminization of Postal Work in Nineteenth-Century France*, by Susan Bachrach

- *Women and the Enlightenment*, by Margaret Hunt, Margaret Jacob, Phyllis Mack, and Ruth Perry, with a Foreword by Ruth Graham

- *The Marriage Bargain: Women and Dowries in European History*, edited by Marion A. Kaplan

- *Industrial Housewives: Women's Social Work in the Factories of Nazi Germany*, by Carola Sachse

Industrial Housewives: Women's Social Work in the Factories of Nazi Germany

Carola Sachse

Translated by
Heide Kiesling and Dorothy Rosenberg
Edited by
Jane Caplan

Copublished by
The Institute for Research in History and The Haworth Press, Inc.

Industrial Housewives: Women's Social Work in the Factories of Nazi Germany has also been published as *Women & History*, Numbers 11/12, 1987.

The Haworth Press, Inc., 12 West 32 Street, New York, NY 10001
EUROSPAN/Haworth, 3 Henrietta Street, London WC2E 8LU England

Library of Congress Cataloging-in-Publication Data

Sachse, Carola, 1951–
    Industrial housewives.

    ''Has also been published as Women & history, numbers 11/12, 1986''—T.p. verso.
    Bibliography: p.
    1. Welfare work in industry—Germany—History. 2. Women—Employment—Germany—History. I. Title.
HD6067.2.G3S23 1986   362.8'5'088042   86-15208
ISBN 0-86656-610-4

Industrial Housewives: Women's Social Work in the Factories of Nazi Germany

Women & History
Numbers 11/12

CONTENTS

Industrial Housewives: Women's Social Work in the Factories of Nazi Germany

Foreword

Jane Caplan

Women's wage work is an essential component of the nation's working life, and the protection and preservation of maternal capacities are the basis for all welfare policies in this area. The German woman should always be conscious of the fact that besides her natural task as the mother of the nation she also serves her people by contributing her labor power in production.

(Gertrud Scholtz-Klink, 1938)[1]

Thus Gertrud Scholtz-Klink, the leader of the NS-Frauenschaft (the National Socialist Women's Group), described the duties of German womanhood in 1938. For those who have the impression that Nazism aimed simply at forcing women back into the home to produce as many baby aryans as possible, Scholtz-Klink's emphatic insistence on wage work outside the home may seem surprising, and also inconsistent with Hitler's own sharp distinction between the public world of men and the private world of women:

. . . her world is her husband, her family, her children, and her house . . . . Providence has entrusted to woman the cares of that world which is peculiarly her own, and only on the basis of this smaller world can the man's world be formed and built up. These two worlds . . . are complementary to each other, they belong together as man and woman belong together.[2]

The image of women's exclusive consignment to the sphere of reproduction is probably one of the most widespread misapprehensions about Nazi Germany, though it does rest on a partial truth. The gist of much Nazi ideology was indeed to assert an essential sociobiological difference between men and women; a difference that was, of course, said to be harmonized in their equally essential complementarity, as the quotation above suggests. This vision of reconciliation also symbolized the fundamental Nazi commitment to the comprehensive social harmony of the *Volksgemeinschaft*, the German national and ethnic community, which was seen as a primary unity to be protected from the discordancy of class and other divisions. But the function of such images is often precisely to celebrate in the ideal what cannot in fact be achieved in the real, and thus to act not as a program for policies but as a substitute for them. In practice, then, women's position and their relationship with men in Nazi Germany tended to elude the simplicities of separate-sphere ideology and to emerge as a series of complex and sometimes contradictory realities.

One of the most important aspects of women's situation was their role in the waged economy, for millions of women did work in the waged sector in the 1930s. In 1933, over 4-1/2 million women could be counted as wage workers in the German economy; in 1939 over five million, and this is without counting the growing numbers of women employed in the white-collar sector.[3] It is with some of the implications of women's work in the industrial sector that Carola Sachse's essay is concerned. Her specific interest is the organization of industrial social work on behalf of women workers in Nazi Germany, and the competition between the different concepts of factory welfare advanced by the employers and by the women's section of the Nazi Labor Front, the compulsory membership organization for workers and employers. Sachse explores the very different priorities of these authorities as they dealt with issues of workforce welfare, and her essay illuminates above all the contrast between the narrowly productivist interests of the employers on the one hand, and the broader social purposes of Nazi interventionism on the other. As an analysis of policies applied to women workers rather than developed by and for them, this essay stands on its own, to be read as an example of how social policy treats women. However, both the immediate context of Nazi Germany and the longer-term development of German social policy are a part of this story which may be unfamiliar to American readers. In this brief introduction I will set out this framework in the hope that this will add to the interest and approachability of the essay itself.

In the nineteenth century, the two leading European industrial nations, Britain and Germany, were also the pioneers of the modern welfare state. By contrast with the contemporary United States, with

its limited sphere of state activity and its cut-throat industrial
competition, industrialism in Europe was more characteristically
accompanied both by growing state intervention in "the social
question," and by employer paternalism (in the provision of
subsidized housing, for example, or the encouragement of workers'
mutual benefit societies). Although philanthropic motives and
sometimes rather innocent visions of class harmony played a part,
both state and employer policies were also frankly self-interested,
serving those who feared the social and political consequences of
unmitigated industrial capitalism. In Germany, these new impulses
combined with the older tradition of the eighteenth-century
Polizeistaat—the interventionist "nightwatchman" state—to stimulate the earliest comprehensive social insurance legislation in
Europe in the 1880s. These laws provided sickness, accident, and
old age insurance, and were intended explicitly to commit workers
to the state as the source of their social welfare, thus distracting
them from the siren-songs of socialism. Whether or not this aim was
achieved in fact, the need for some such stratagem was strongly felt
among employers and state officials alike, as a response to the
extraordinarily rapid progress of industrial development in Germany
in the late nineteenth century.[4]

The question of conditions of employment was a part of this
concern. Factory regulation began seriously in the 1860s; the first
codification of protective legislation was adopted in 1891, and was
extended and amended several times before the First World War.
As in most nineteenth-century factory legislation, in Germany, too,
official concern for the regulation of hours of work, accident
prevention, working conditions, and so on was intimately con-
nected with anxieties about the moral and eugenic consequences of
women's work. Thus the 1891 act stipulated, for example, that
factories under its jurisdiction were to be laid out in accordance not
only with the principles of accident prevention, but also with the
maintenance of "morality" (*Sittlichkeit*) including, for instance,
the provision of sex-segregated washing and changing facilities.
Measures like this recognized the increasing employment of women
in the factory labor force: by 1907 there were over a million women
industrial workers. Although the conditions of the much larger
numbers of female domestics and home-workers were legislatively
ignored for far longer, there were vigorous contemporary debates
about women's work and protective legislation, in which, of
course, both bourgeois and proletarian feminists also took part. By

1896, social democrat feminists were on the whole committed to the principle of protective legislation, while bourgeois feminists were divided on whether this might be disadvantageous to their own demands for equal employment opportunities in the professions. It was at about the same time that the first female factory inspectors were appointed: by 1906 there were 16 women among the total of 350, and 26 by 1910.[5] Women as workers were thus the object of a variety of policies before the war. In addition, as Sachse points out, employers anxious to secure a stable and reliable labor force in heavily "male" industries, such as steel-making or coal-mining, were also interested in promoting domestic stability and comfort by various provisions aimed at women as wives and homemakers.

By 1914, then, the framework for the later factory welfare policies examined by Sachse had already been established, and included a number of different elements. The state had intervened early in industrial social policy, at least partly as a politically precautionary measure, while proclaiming its aim to be the "protection of national labor" (*Schutz der nationalen Arbeit*). State and employer paternalism might converge to some degree where the needs of labor discipline and social stability were interrelated, but many employers were clearly reluctant to concede a right of national state intervention beyond a certain point—that point being the individual firm's calculation of its profitability. In these circumstances, employers might prefer to make their own social provisions, if any; they were certainly not going to bow to invocations of any national interest. When women were part of these calculations, they might figure either as members of the waged workforce or as the wives or mothers or daughters of male workers (sometimes as both, no doubt). If the former, they were more likely to be employed in sectors like the consumer industries, where employers tended to show little interest in paternalist social policy (since labor formed such a high proportion of production costs), than in heavy and extractive industry, where employers supplemented state paternalism with their own schemes to ensure labor discipline through the family. On the whole, as Sachse argues, before the First World War employers' welfare efforts were directed more at women's family than workforce roles. And finally, state social policies had begun to elicit the formation of a new profession of female factory inspectors, whom we can see to some extent as the forerunners of the trained women welfare officers in the interwar period, discussed in detail in Sachse's essay.

Before 1914, women workers did not form a very large proportion of the total industrial labor force. In 1913, 1.4 million women were employed in enterprises of nine or more workers, compared with 5.4 million men. But during the war this picture changed, as millions of men were conscripted into the armed services, and women were drawn into industry to take their place. By 1918, the comparable figures showed 3.8 million men, and 2.1 million women: thus women's industrial employment had increased both absolutely and proportionately. The figures for women employed by the heavy industrial and armaments firm of Krupp illustrate this dramatically: where women had been 3.2 percent of its workforce in 1913, they were 37.6 percent in 1918.[6] It was in this new context that welfare work on behalf of women as workers (and not as the dependents of male workers) began to expand, as Sachse shows in the first section of her essay. What is worth emphasizing is that these wartime provisions were not launched by employers on the whole, but were developed on state initiative; and, as in other aspects of the war effort, the state enjoyed the active cooperation of the less radical women's and worker's organizations. The wartime emergency thus brought previously antagonistic groups into a form of alliance. Although this was to break down at the end of the war, some of the same impulses to collaboration were almost certainly at work again in the 1930s, among those (not all of them Nazis) who accepted the view that German recovery from the depression was now an emergency issue.

At the end of the war, women were squeezed back out of the "male" industrial sectors in Germany as elsewhere. However, women's wage work began to increase in the 1920s in the newer sectors of white-collar and light industrial employment.[7] This shift in the structure of production and employment was experienced in other industrial economies, but in Germany it was also accompanied by an acceleration of industrial rationalization which was unparalleled in Europe. America was probably the only capitalist economy which embraced rationalization to a similar extent. Rationalization affected not only the production processes themselves, but also such aspects as management, office organization, the selection and deployment of workers and so on. The existing paternalism of

German industrial management was now met by a new tendency to adopt "modern" management and personnel policies, which to some extent enjoyed the cooperation of labor unions as well. Sachse shows how both the older paternalism and the newer rationalization movement influenced the development of industrial social work in the 1920s. Two patterns can be distinguished: the "Ruhr" or heavy industry model, which still concentrated on women as members of the male workers' families; and the "Bielefeld" or light industry model, which was directed at improving the productivity of an unskilled female labor force. By the time the National Socialist regime took over in 1933, the German economy had been profoundly disrupted by four years of deep depression and crisis, but it was in the context of these two tendencies, with their linkages to different sectors and concepts of production, that the new regime approached the issues of women's wage work and social policy.

The Nazi period is the focus of Sachse's essay, and I will not attempt to summarize her arguments here; her aims and approach are in any case set out very clearly in the introduction. However, I would like to highlight a couple of the points which may be less familiar to anyone who hasn't followed the recent literature on the history of National Socialism—of which, as always, there seems to be a never-ending stream.

Sachse's essay is written in the light of two long-standing debates about the structure of recent German history. The more far-reaching of these raises questions about the placement of the National Socialist period in modern German history since unification and industrialization in the nineteenth century. On the one hand, this seems to be a history full of ruptures and discontinuities—the establishment of the empire in 1871, its overthrow by the republican revolution in 1918, the turbulent brevity of the Nazi period from 1933 to 1945, the division and divergence of East and West Germany since then. But on the other hand, this apparent discontinuity seems to be contradicted by the durability of some aspects of Germany's fundamental economic and social structures, and by the recurrence of certain basic national objectives, such as the continental imperialism which was part of German aims in both world wars.

Some historians have argued that this contradiction reflects an objective and peculiarly German historical incongruence: the contrast between Germany's economic "modernization" as an advanced capitalist system, and its social and political "backwardness", which long precluded the eclipse of aristocratic feudal power and the development of a fully democratic parliamentary state. In this view, economic modernization passed over certain social groups—especially the aristocracy, and the rural and urban petty bourgeoisie—and cemented a conservative alliance between them against the forces of change, represented in particular by the working-class movement. Similarly, even the bourgeoisie is said to have been "feudalized," in the sense of accepting the values of the old landowning class instead of developing values and aspirations appropriate to its own social and economic position.

Thus, in this view, the conflicts of both 1918 and 1933 can be seen as evidence of the ruling groups' intractibility when challenged by liberal and socialist forces. The Nazi regime itself could be seen partly as a bungled attempt by the old elites and ruling groups to rescue themselves from crisis, in an alliance with the only force strong enough to save them in an era of mass politics—the Nazi movement. These interpretations have, however, been rejected by other historians, on the grounds that they apply an eclectic model of modernization drawn mainly from Anglo-American experience. To test Germany against this, and find it wanting, is not so much a verdict on German history as on the inappropriateness of the model in the first place. German history, in this view, is but one specific form of industrial growth and social change which should be judged on its own terms. It should not be forced into a mold of expected development, and its successive crises and ruptures should be seen as evidence of basic shifts in power relations, not of immutable conflicts between fixed social and political groups.[8]

The second debate is more circumscribed: the nature of the Nazi regime itself. In the past, and especially to its contemporaries, the "Third Reich" seemed an archetype of totalitarian uniformity and efficiency, manipulating its subjects in pursuit of long-chosen goals. With more historical perspective and detailed research, however, has come the recognition that the regime was a hotbed of contradictions and rivalries. These were not just personal quarrels over the spoils of power, but real conflicts that in part derived from the persistent pluralism at the economic and social level, despite the massive concentration of political authority. Political pluralism may have been abolished after 1933, but the social antagonisms that it had carried were merely played out at a different level, inside the structure of the ostensibly unitary state.[9] Research into almost any aspect of the regime tends to reveal widely divergent interests among policy-makers within the regime, as well as disagreements with outsiders, as Sachse shows in her discussion of NSDAP and employer debates on social policy.

Both of these wider historiographical debates inform Sachse's approach to her specific subject. For example, what elements of the old paternalism can be detected in industrialists' espousal of industrial welfare work, or how far was it a highly modern response to the new "problem" of women's wage work? Was the German Labor Front more traditionalist or modernizing in its own approach to the question? What happened when a vigorous eugenicism was injected into state policies for women? These questions are not merely of antiquarian interest: the trapping of women into the "natural" and timeless category of motherhood alongside their more obviously contingent roles in industry is very much a concern of contemporary women. Moreover, women's history of the kind presented here can do more than simply contribute to the state of knowledge about the past and the present. It can also act to redefine categories and boundaries. Thus "continuity" for women may look very different from continuity for states or political practices or economic processes: It is clear, for instance, that similar practices in respect of sex and gender are in fact compatible with very different political and social systems. The whole debate about capitalism and patriarchy has made this (if nothing else) clear, and Sachse's essay offers us some provocative illustrations of it.

In the context of her article, we might want to see the 1920s and 1930s in Germany as actually very similar in the ongoing concern among industrialists and the state to resolve some of the contradictions raised by women's increasing involvement in both productive and reproductive, waged and unwaged labor.[10] This remains an issue in many industrialized countries, though it is noteworthy that the percentage of West German women in the waged labor force has been more static than elsewhere.[11] Current feminist work on Nazi Germany is also placing new emphasis on the complex relationships between gender, class, and race as axes of exploitation and subordination.[12] Carola Sachse's work adds to our knowledge of specific sites of subordination and suggests how some interconnections are established. The extremity of the context—a nation in the grip of an oppressive and uniquely inhumane fascist dictatorship, and then engulfed in a ferocious war—may be unusual, but the concerns of policy were not. The realm of welfare continues to be one of the most fruitful ways to raise and investigate the problems of women's situation in capitalist society—and whatever else it was, Nazi Germany was also that.

ENDNOTES

1. Gertrud Scholtz-Klink, *Die Frau im Dritten Reich, Eine Dokumentation* (Tübingen, 1978), 320.

2. Hitler's speech to women at the Nuremberg NSDAP rally, 8 September 1934, in Norman H. Baynes, ed., *The Speeches of Adolf Hitler April 1922-August 1939*, (London, 1942): 528.

3. Dörte Winkler, *Frauenarbeit im 'Dritten Reich'* (Hamburg, 1977), 195.

4. See for example W.O. Henderson, *The Rise of German Industrial Power 1834-1914* (London, 1975), Part 3.

5. See Heinz Niggemann, *Emanzipation zwischen Sozialismus und Feminismus. Die Sozialdemokratische Frauenbewegung im Kaiserreich* (Wuppertal, 1981), 134–42.

6. Ludwig Preller, *Sozialpolitik in der Weimarer Republik* (reprint ed., Düsseldorf, 1978), 7–8.

7. See Renate Bridenthal, "Beyond *Kinder, Küche, Kirche*: Weimar Women at Work," *Central European History* 6 (1973), 148–166.

8. For a discussion of these issues, see David Blackbourn and Geoff Eley, *The Peculiarities of German History: Bourgeois Society and Politics in Nineteenth Century Germany* (Oxford, 1984).

9. See for example Martin Broszat, *The Hitler State* (London/New York, 1981).

10. See Annemarie Tröger, "The Creation of a Female Assembly-Line Proletariat," in Renate Bridenthal, Atina Grossmann, and Marion Kaplan, eds., *When Biology became Destiny: Women in Weimar and Nazi Germany* (New York, 1984).

11. See Angelika Willms, "The Socialization of Women's Work: The Case of Germany, 1882-1979," VASMA Working Paper No. 19 (Mannheim, 1981); also published in K. Hvidfeldt, K. Jørgensen and R. Nielsen, eds., *Strategies for Integrating Women into the Labour Market* (Copenhagen, 1982), 121–144.

12. For sources in English, see the essay collection in note 10 and also Gisela Bock, "Racism and Sexism in Nazi Germany: Motherhood, Compulsory Sterilization, and the State," *Signs; A Journal of Woman in Culture and Society*, vol. 8, no. 3 (Spring 1983): 400–21.

Introduction

In an essay published in 1926, economist and social activist
Frieda Wunderlich called social welfare workers in German manu-
facturing plants the "housewives of industry."[1] This was an apt
label: industrial social workers were concerned with the orderliness,
cleanliness, and pleasantness of conditions in workers' homes and
occasionally provided a potted geranium to adorn a factory
windowsill. Social workers were responsible for the "purely human" aspects of industry: they helped new female workers become
acquainted with the factory and introduce themselves to their co-
workers, and they smoothed conflicts among workers as well as
between labor and management. They dealt with workers' problems
not only in the workplace but also in private, and family matters.
Industrial social workers tried to create a conflict-free industrial
climate, sustained by a system of courteous yet binding human
relations.[2] In order to maintain the strict neutrality they believed this
goal required, social workers thought it necessary to work behind
the scenes, suppress their own personalities, and forego recognition
of their achievements. Who was better adapted to do this than
women?

The industrial welfare worker may not expect that what she
has achieved will become visible. Rather what will come to
light is the fact that the good and right thing is being done. For
this reason she must seek out opportunities to increase cooperation among a wider circle, especially among supervisors.
She will find this much easier if she demonstrates a sense of
trust and appeals to others' better nature. She must always be
mindful of the responsibility she shares to strengthen the trust
between supervisors and the members of the workshops. She
would therefore do well to take every opportunity to allow the
supervisors to convey any good news. For example: a desired
transfer to another location or the approval of a recreational
leave.[3]

Industrial welfare work, introduced in Germany at the turn of the century, adapted itself easily to the National Socialist version of the capitalist system, its philosophy that the "industrial community" is the seed from which springs the "community of the German People," and its conception of social policy. Under the Nazi regime, entrepreneurs became "plant managers," and were urged to adopt immediately a welfare system that National Socialists believed would inspire loyalty in all workers, male and female.[4] But "industrial social work" was also regarded as a women's issue, and was, in fact, the focal point of the National Socialist program for women workers. With a tireless expenditure of propaganda the National Socialists laid claim to the field of social work as their own invention. They extolled it as an advance in industrial social policy and as a solution to the problem of women in industry.[5]

This study traces industrial social work from its inception through the Nazi period, examines its continuities and discontinuities, and assesses the effect on the industrial welfare system of developments within National Socialism.[6] With regard to the scholarly controversy over the political character of National Socialism, this study adopts the position that it was not a monolithic power structure. Rather, it was a polycratic regime which continually had to accept compromises and adjustments.[7] Within this framework the study examines the role of women in industrial social work and labor relations, the attitudes of various groups toward the proper relations between industry and government, and the well-documented relationship between industrialists and the German Labor Front (Deutsche Arbeitsfront, or DAF), the National Socialist organization that replaced the outlawed labor unions.[8] This study, of course, focuses on women and their work. Because of their special problems as workers, women had long been the particular concern of industrial social policy. All branches of industry were confronted with the fact that women were not only factory workers, but also, and primarily, housewives, wives, mothers, daughters, sisters, and aunts. In addition to themselves, they had to look after other family members. To help women reconcile their conflicting roles in the best interests of the family, industry, and national community, industry and government called on the services of professional "good angels," the industrial social workers.

Industrial social work centered on the burden and the management of the double workload for women workers. It was the point at which wage work and housework by women, the industrial and extra-industrial production by both sexes, the factory, and family, came together. Overseeing the dual work of women became more important as women were shifted from the periphery to the center of industrial production and had to be made more productive members of the workforce. Government and party authorities and various branches of industry proposed policies for accomplishing their goals in this sphere and for setting the political priorities according to which they would be adopted. In the continual process of policy formation, each of these interests also sought to establish its own position.[9]

This study essentially follows the chronology by which industrial social work evolved as an aspect of industrial social policy in Germany. It then focuses on two distinct models of industrial social work, which were formulated in the 'twenties and gradually put into practice: The Bielefeld, or light industry model; and the Ruhr, or heavy industry model. This is followed by a discussion of the concept of industrial social work as presented by the Nazi Reich Women's Leader (Reichsfrauenführerin), Gertrud Scholtz-Klink, and in National Socialist publications.[10] The diverse interests of state and party organizations will be analyzed as well as the concerns of industry with respect to its social and political relationship with the female labor force. In discussions of industrial social work, the DAF acted as the representative of Nazi industrial policy. Ranged against the state and party "line" was the Reichsgruppe Industrie, the organization of German industrialists in the Nazi system, which represented the interests of industrial entrepreneurs in the Reich Economic Council. While the Nazis continually put forward their own proposals, industry attempted to avoid any substantive discussion of policy content. In the formal area of principle and regulation, industry sought to maintain its autonomy.

The focus of this study is industrial social work as a policy executed by those with authority over women and their labor; it does not approach it from the viewpoint of either the social workers or their clients. This is primarily due to the nature of the source material.[11] After the abolition by the Nazis of their professional associations, the women's and workers' movements could neither organize nor speak, nor could their members as individuals openly express ideas too far divergent from official positions. The same was true of the social workers' clients, working women and workers' wives. Thus it is almost impossible to make clear assertions about the intentions of the social workers in industry or the extent to which they made use of available opportunities to assist their clients, hampered as they were by the directives of their industrial superiors, party and DAF functionaries, and still more highly placed authorities.

Industrial social work developed in the 1920s as an aspect of the industrial social policy that had been evolving according to the strategies of employers. After the first World War, in the light of changing social, economic, and technical production requirements, industrial authorities reorganized and adjusted their traditional industrial welfare measures to the political restrictions of a more developed and more socially interventionist state. Technical changes in the industrial labor process and other considerations led employers to experiment with methods for more integrated industrial policy, including "yellow" (company) unions, plant newspapers, and plant-wide personnel management. Labor relations consequently took on a new aspect, and the effect on the social and family relationships of the labor force created a larger role for welfare work in the industrial policy of big business.[12]

In the 'twenties, industrial social work was discussed by employer and labor unions and in several large firms it was put into practice and added to existing labor relations measures. Industrial social work was also adopted as an educational project. Women's Social Work Schools developed training programs in the new methods for industrial welfare workers. For the labor sciences (labor physiology, ergonomics, labor psychology, psychotechnics) industrial social work was *the* innovative measure in industrial social policy of the 'twenties. It was discussed in numerous national and international meetings and conferences and with great frequency in influential newspapers.[13]

In the National Socialist period industrial social work was thoroughly institutionalized. The employment of "industrial social workers," as they were called by the National Socialists (previously they had been known variously as plant welfare workers, social workers, or social industrial workers) especially in industries employing a female labor force, was a substantial demand which the DAF, as the self-proclaimed representative of all working Germans, presented to employers. Although no breakdown exists for the Nazi period to show exactly which companies employed industrial social workers and it is not possible to estimate the number of their female clients, we do know that the number of industrial social workers rose to 3,000 during the Second World War.[14]

Chapter One:
The Beginnings
of Industrial Social Work

Serious employer interest in family welfare dates from the 1870s, when it first became clear that Germany had definitely shifted from an agrarian to an industrial economy and that the process of industrial production was being transformed. Enterprises which had been based on the traditional model of craft production in workshops were being consolidated into a more rigidly structured system of unified production based on the division of labor. Even with the dramatic increase in the number of unskilled personnel a minimum level of training was required for workers, but in the new environment other qualities, such as punctuality, dependability, and the ability to adjust to discipline, became more important. Other significant developments in this period were an apparently unlimited influx of new and highly exploitable workers from the countryside, the growth of labor unions, and the establishment of a government social security system.

Against this background, conflicting expectations of the women's work force emerged. According to the bourgeois domestic standards of Prussian state and educational authorities, the nuclear family—breadwinner, housewife, and child—was the basic model for a stable society, as exemplified, for instance, in the recently established social security system.[15] Yet the fact that industry also required women's labor power was not seriously (or at any rate successfully) called into question by any sector of German society.

Industry exercised different forms of control over women, depending on their marital and occupational status. Some were brought into the factory and in effect housed in barracks: for example, some factories drew their female workers from local workhouses, educational institutions, or prisons and some even had these directly attached to their premises.[16] Workers' wives received home economic training, which from the employers' point of view killed two birds with one stone. First, thrifty running of the household made possible the adequate reproduction of the worker family on a low wage level. Second, the women thus trained became able to earn additional income through ironing, needlework, or housecleaning, which was funneled into the household upkeep.

Industry also was motivated to establish family welfare programs for female employees who continued to work after marriage. The focus here was on training "their own" women in how to combine housework and work outside the home without creating friction in the workplace. Employers were now more interested in employing married women: their earlier reliance on hiring women who could be housed in barracks, women from the fringes of society and single women, had given factory labor an air of disreputability. Industry was now interested in recruiting a more stable class of women more likely to have the desired qualities of punctuality, diligence, and loyalty. Such women, if single, would doubtless be marriageable or at least desirous of marrying, and more likely to welcome employment in a factory with a welfare system and without barracks.

The contradictions in the demands on women's labor sharpened during a second period of industrial rationalization around 1905, and during the First World War, the situation came to a dramatic head, completely surprising those responsible for it. Mothers in vast numbers were forced to work in factories without any provision for their children; factory welfare workers and consultants of the women's office could give them only the scantest help, and many of the children died.[17]

Still, industrial social work experienced a dramatic upswing during the First World War. This occurred to a large extent through government action, as a result of the increased employment of female workers and complaints about their unwillingness to work, low productivity, and poor discipline. The Center for Women's Labor (Frauenarbeitszentrale, or FAZ) in the War Office, under the leadership of Marie-Elisabeth Lüders, began to "organize the mobilization of women by women" in order to stimulate "readiness for work," "ability to work," and "steadiness at work."[18]

To achieve these aims, the FAZ pushed for the appointment of factory welfare workers in industrial plants to act so to speak, as its footsoldiers. As a result, in 1917, government controlled industries employing women were required by the War Ministry to hire factory welfare workers; private arms manufacturers also had to comply with this regulation under threat of losing their contracts.[19] This incorporation of welfare work into personnel policy was not

motivated by humanitarianism or considerations of profitability. It
was the result of pressure from above, where a few women from the
"bourgeois" or "organized" women's movement were in positions
of influence.[20]

The factory social service workers were trained in four-to-eight-
week courses given by the regional branches of the War Office or
the Women's Sections or Women's Labor Centrals attached to
them, which were generally led by women. The courses were
frequently offered in cooperation with Women's Social Work
Schools which had been growing more numerous since 1916.[21] The
participants in these continuing education courses were selected in
an "unusually strict screening" by "morally superior personages"
from the "upper social classes," already trained in social work.
They introduced their students to the basics of industrial hygiene,
industrial safety, and insurance law. In addition, the participants
worked briefly in a factory "in order to be better able to judge the
lines between 'should,' 'will,' and 'can,' for women workers from
their own experience of the work, and to make suggestions for
facilitating the workers' tasks or trying out new work routines."
Only rarely were trainees chosen by women workers from their own
ranks, and these were "in enterprises with an especially elevated
workforce."[22]

By July 1918, 789 factory social service workers were responsible for approximately 733,000 women workers in 1,176 factories,
i.e., about 35 percent of the female labor force.[23] These female
factory workers were, however, no longer predominantly single,
childless, young or adolescent as before the war. Now, increasingly, married women, mothers, and women with dependents to
care for were coming into the factories, mostly out of financial
necessity. Many had relocated to the location of a new armaments
factory. This change in the labor force created new problems for the
industrial welfare workers, who now had to provide support services
for factory work, housework, and childcare. They organized shopping services, ran errands to government offices, established day
care centers, and, where necessary, arranged further social services
for the workers' families. At the same time, they attempted to
familiarize the women with the factory workplace and monitored
working conditions in the factory, especially hygiene, sanitation and
also, to some extent, the physical demands of work. They also took
the time to respond personally to the women and their problems.[24]

Immediately after the war, most firms dismissed the industrial welfare workers, who had more or less been forced upon them, as well as the married women who were now suddenly regarded as "double earners," i.e., second wage earners in the family. A few companies, however, retained the social workers and in some areas, for example in the electrical industry and in the Ruhr mining industry, the plant welfare system, as it was now frequently called, was even expanded—this time, however, under the sole direction of the employer, who more and more frequently sought out graduates of the Women's Social Work Schools.[25]

In the turbulent postwar period policy makers, social reformers, and businessmen began to regard the ordinary working-class family as society's panacea for the decadence of youth. It could also be an instrument for improving general health conditions and a bulwark against worker radicalism and the resulting decline in productivity. Working-class marriages were especially encouraged and, for whatever reasons, more marriages took place. It was these women aged twenty to thirty, now married and often with small children, who proved most efficient under the specialized demands of the assembly line. And because of the widespread impoverishment of German society through war and inflation, many of them, especially those of the lower classes, were forced into the factories in order to save their children.[26] Social and economic conditions thus made it increasingly difficult to avoid conflicting labor demands on women by splitting the potential female labor force into full time housewives and workers. More and more women had to furnish housework, childcare, and factory work at the same time. These women were the challenge for the industrial social policy of the 'twenties.

MANAGEMENT VIEWS
INDUSTRIAL SOCIAL WORK

For employers, problems in industrial social work varied according to factors specific to different regions, industries, and branches of production. Regional factors included the size, composition, and structure of the labor markets from which an industry recruited its work force. Industry-specific factors relevant to social work policy were the absolute size of the body of employees, the composition of personnel, and the availability of a regional labor force. Significant variation in the composition of the labor force included marital status (the proportion of married and unmarried laborers, the number of children), the proportion of resident and newly arrived or recruited labor, and their ethnic affiliation. Branch-specific influences on industrial social policy included the composition of the labor force, both in terms of relative status (ratio of blue-collar and white-collar workers) and qualifications (skilled and unskilled), and according to age and sex.

The firms that were most active in family welfare (and which were later to become involved in discussions with the DAF) employed hundreds of thousands of workers among them: Vereinigte Stahlwerke, Siemens, Krupp, IG Farben. With their commitment to scientific management, all matters affecting production were seen as economically calculable cost factors. Family welfare was, for them, something that could be costed according to these principles of industrial economy.

Several of the firms dominated their labor markets or were almost the only employers: for example, Krupp in Essen, IG Farben/Basf in Ludwigshafen, IG Farben/Bayer in Leverkusen, and to a much more limited degree, Siemens in Berlin-Siemensstadt. This meant that these companies were dependent on a specific working population from one generation to the next and that, therefore, a long term and well-planned policy in relation to the available work force was desirable. In many locations the industry-based welfare (hospitals, convalescent homes, kindergartens, leisure facilities) could be incorporated with the bulk of municipal contributions. For other companies particular strategies were indicated by local conditions; for example, to strengthen their position in the local labor market (e.g., Merck in Darmstadt), to recruit a specialized and hitherto unavailable type of labor (e.g., Oetker in Bielefeld), or to turn a labor force recruited from outside into long term, settled residents, as did some textile factories in Westphalia.[27]

The first question in determining the type of family welfare system adopted and the method of operation was whether it was to deal with men, women, or both. The iron and steel mining industries employed an almost exclusively male workforce up to the first years of the Second World War. In regions such as the Ruhr, the wives of these men were occupied primarily in the home, although when necessary they pursued some form of income-supplementing work. Thus, mining and steel employers had scarcely been confronted with the "modern double burden" placed on workers' wives and saw no reason to depart from their long-standing, family-oriented programs, which had characteristically developed in the Ruhr area.

But things appeared somewhat different in regions less dominated by a single industry and for those firms with an exclusively male labor force. Here, employers had to reckon with the fact that the wives of their workers themselves worked, assembling vacuum cleaners or sewing uniforms, and were away from their homes for up to ten or twelve hours a day. In these cases, employers could try to convince the women, or better still their husbands, of the impropriety of this. But ultimately it was a question of money. Plant welfare workers could be sent in to try to persuade women to take up some kind of work that was more "appropriate to their family responsibilities" or to convince them that they could manage without some of their income (i.e., their own wage) if they only ran their households more rationally (i.e., more economically).

The interest of industry in the female laborers it employed was entirely different. In this case, the increasing marriage rate of working women and their consequent withdrawal from the workforce was undesirable, since their labor was needed. However, there was no way to abolish this socially valuable institution. These companies were forced to institute a "modern" home economy program for their women workers which would save the women's time and strength for factory work. They also made available institutional aid, which minimized the absenteeism due to family concerns.

Companies with mixed (male and female) workers encountered still more conflicts. An industry's publicly-proclaimed commitment to the orderly working-class family was hardly convincing if, at the same time, it employed married women and mothers of small children, requiring them to be outside the home during shifts of eight to ten hours. Industrial social work could not get away with simply balancing the contradictions of the female work force by means of philanthropic self-interest; rather, it had to fully legitimize women's dual burden as *the* modern form of working-class family life.

The industrial welfare workers saw themselves as a mediating agency between management and labor, and this was their intended function. But they were, in fact, a part of personnel management and directly under the control of factory executives. In these circumstances, acquiring the trust of the workers and their families, the pre-condition for a successful industrial welfare system as defined by the employer, was naturally a delicate matter. If they were vocal representatives of their clients, they could very quickly lose their jobs; if they spoke as supervisors, they could face suspicion and rejection by the workers. Management, of course, was aware of this dilemma, and allowed the plant welfare officers a certain discretion in maintaining confidentiality concerning the personal relationships and problems of their clients. It also did not contradict the interests of management to allow, in closely controlled individual cases, the workers or their families to be granted carefully dispensed assistance. In practice the lines between material support, welfare work, and control and discipline were fluid.[28] In the final analysis, the resolution of this quandary always rested with the individual welfare worker. Employers did not intend to bring women's advocates, onto the factory council, and did not regard welfare workers as such. Contemporary sources stress the harmony between factory management and plant welfare officers.

Chapter Two:
Factory Family Welfare in the 1920s

In the 1920s, for the first time, industrial family welfare systems were developed in Germany under the sole control of employers, without any direct intervention in their social and educational principles by the state, local government, churches, or labor unions. However, these systems did not evolve in isolation from contemporary debates about social policy and pedagogical principles: industrial welfare workers themselves, trained as they were in the Women's Social Work Schools, channeled into the industrial sphere the social welfare ideas of the Weimar Period.

At this time there were about 100 or 150 women employed as factory social service workers.[29] They were now beginning to be known as "industrial welfare workers," a term that expressed the changing emphasis in social work. Before the war, factory social work had been chiefly a matter of looking after young and single women workers during their work and leisure time and training them in domesticity and family life in order to prepare them for their future responsibilities as housewives. But by demonstrating the contradictory nature of the women's dual labor in household and factory, the war had made the integration of this duality the object of factory social service work. In the view of social policy makers, the biggest threat arising from women's double labor was not the overtaxing of women workers, but the destabilization of the family, which critics believed to be the result of women's employment outside the home. The central object of the efforts of all industrial welfare workers now was not so much the individual worker in the factory as the domestic sphere of the working-class family. Their objective was to combat "want, sickness, moral neglect, despair, and radicalism. . . . at their source," believed to be "primarily in the family."[30]

Welfare workers regarded the family household as an "economic and social factor of utmost significance."[31] That the work of women was decisive was apparent not only to the plant welfare officers but to the company management as well: "The best income cannot help a family to get on in the world if the wife is not a good manager and the money slips through her fingers.''[32]

Good management generally meant coping with scarcity and utilizing leftovers. Therefore, the welfare workers instructed women in "how one can still make something decent out of old clothing and that the same can be applied to food: how to cook something decent and tasty with a certain amount of variety and without great expenditure.''[33] This was, without question, a self-serving version of the social-pedagogical principle of helping those who help themselves. Rather than pay adequate wages, the firms preferred to show women how they could use their labor within the home more efficiently to keep within the existing family budget. To do this, employers again took advantage of women's labor, namely, that of the industrial welfare workers.[34]

Many firms carried on the tradition of factory-owned sewing and mending schools, which had existed here and there since the 1880s. Under the direction of the plant welfare officers, these firms also established schools of home economics which held evening courses for women workers and workers' wives. Full-time two-year programs were provided for workers' daughters who had finished grade school.[35] The course offerings ranged from "sheet ironing," infant care, and educational precepts to "citizenship." The schools of instruction made heavy demands on the students, seeking to "involve the whole young person through systematic work.''[36]

Training and continuing education in domestic economy were part of the standard program of all industrial welfare workers. Even when they were not always able to conduct their own classes, the social workers were still able to visit the workers' homes. During these visits they could observe household management and give advice to improve the women's housekeeping. Now and then they would even provide tangible support—although money was practically never given. The women probably accepted these visits more frequently with suspicion than with good will.[37]

The home economics schools in the Ruhr coal, iron, and steel industries were the most numerous and provided the most extensive course offerings.[38] There too, the German Institute for Technical Labor Training (Deutsches Institut für Technische Arbeitsschulung, or DINTA) propagated its "factory community" efforts most widely. Interested in rationalizing women's housework to save on wages, it attempted to gain influence over the workers' entire domestic life and to integrate their families into the "factory family." DINTA went so far as to demand that the public social work system should be substantially replaced by welfare facilities provided by each factory and that these should be as far as possible, self-supporting. "Our basic principle is not to give, but to work for," as one plant welfare officer put it.[39]

That the idea of a family welfare system found an especially favorable response in the Ruhr district was due to the area's long tradition of industrial social policy, together with Ruhr employers' active rejection of the state and municipal social policy which had been fought for by both the workers' and the women's movements. The fact that the inhabitants of the industrial region represented a "colorful multiplicity of nationalities without common manners and customs" had helped this paternalistic tradition to survive.

Welfare workers reported that Ruhr workers lived in "repulsively ugly" industrial towns in company housing, usually distinguished by "dreary uniformity," and "gloominess and neglect." Family life was far indeed from the model envisioned by DINTA, the Ruhr employers, and the plant welfare workers:

> The industrial man is hardly acquainted with a firm set of domestic rules, knows no integration into a common family life. Club life and Party confiscate the soul of the husband and remove him from the family both after work and on Sunday, his day off. Movie theaters, dance halls, coffee houses with jazz music and their like lure youths from the family circle and help to shatter it. While few of our miners' wives have sought work outside of their homes, there are not many of them who have an internal means of defense against the obtrusiveness of their surroundings and routine; or many capable of offering, through their depth of motherliness, a counterbalance to all of these destructive influences or the noise and soot in our region. We have therefore dedicated our industrial welfare system to these educational goals: cultivation of national character, the strengthening of a sense of family, and the elevation of family morals. We will endeavor to mobilize all forces for the family from the family.[40]

With this goal, the industrial welfare went beyond the technical and economic problems of the organization of housework. Now it undertook the battle against "proletarian hopelessness which stifled initiative, independence, and the joy of living.''[41] Its starting point was the women:

> In the lower classes the wife dominates and directs the husband in an unexpected way. She is a tireless and sharp-tongued agitator who can be reached by no penal law and whose influence no rational counter-argument can neutralize. She does not shrink from the strongest forms of incitement to lead the way in a struggle and to call her husband a coward. And it is just this appeal to his male pride or, in a negative sense, the expression of doubt in his ability to exist and to succeed, which hurls the man into the struggle.[42]

Welfare workers taught that wives should have not behave like political agitators to their husbands and convert their dissatisfactions into an offensive: rather, it was their "duty as mothers and nurturers" to be conciliators—to prevent their husbands from missing work, keep them away from alcohol, encourage their thrift, and push for "the acquisition of a home of their own."

Since industry was "keenly interested in fostering an efficient and reliable working class," industrial welfare workers urged women to become "happy and cheerful creatures whose very natures encourage their families and the husbands who come home in the evening tired and in need of rest.''[43] Industrial welfare workers also tried to "cultivate taste and a sense of color and form" by showing the women how they could decorate their homes with a "brightly colored afghan and a few flowers." Although workers' wives had no objections to such programs, they did not consider themselves solely responsible for the comfort of their homes, and demanded that appropriate "fathers' nights" be organized for the domestic instruction of their husbands. These were in fact instituted.[44]

It was good policy for the workers' wives, to present a carefully managed household and well-groomed children to the industrial welfare worker on her home visits. Obtaining emergency benefits could depend on this. The West Mills of the Amalgamated Steelworks Corporation (August Thyssen Mills) kept detailed benefit application forms on file, including a complicated point system which gave a plus point for a "very clean" household and "good" childcare, but assigned two minus points if things were "untidy.''[45]

Thus, an elaborate plan for the proletarian household and family lay behind the industrial welfare system as practiced in the 1920s. The central point was the labor of women as housewives, which was to be rationalized, just as the industrial labor of both men and women had been. The plan started with the thrifty, "productive" utilization of wages. This would guarantee the reproduction of the labor force at low wages and reduce the necessity of paying supplemental benefits, since thrifty housewives would open savings accounts and workers' families could help themselves.[46] The rationalization of domestic work allowed time and energy for making family life pleasant, with a cozy home, well-behaved and well-groomed children, and a contented, untroubled husband.[47] Industry's economic interests would also be advanced by the domestic program's elimination of financial worries for the bread-winner, and the resultant improved productivity of the male work force. Employers believed it was "a decisive factor for the working man . . . whether he comes to work full of domestic worries, ill-humored, and worn out, or whether he comes from an orderly household."[48]

Chapter Three:
The Bielefeld Model
of Industrial Social Work

The Bielefeld, or light-industry model of industrial social work, statistically insignificant in the 1920s, assumed great importance in 1933, when it was adopted by the Women's Bureau of the German Labor Front (DAF), influenced by a Bielefeld proponent, Ilse Ganzert, at that time still a member of a free trade union, and developed into the centerpiece of the Nazi policy for women in the factories.[49] The Bielefeld model differed in one significant way from family welfare-oriented industrial social work: it was directed toward exactly those women whom the Ruhr employers had excluded from their factory welfare systems—persons with whom the factory welfare workers expected to encounter "insurmountable difficulties" and who were therefore left to the municipal welfare system. These less promising clients, such as "the girls who have arrived as immigrants by the hundreds and are housed in barracks," were left to their own devices by the Ruhr system, even when they "very quickly [became] a public nuisance."[50] Because of the long-term unemployment of the 1920s, the employers could afford to reject these "inferior" workers, who were by nature especially in need of care and assistance.[51]

Nonetheless, there were still firms, especially in the textile industry, and whole regions which were dependent upon this "inferior," and cheap labor. These were the firms which then hired industrial social workers:

> A linen spinning mill which had located in Westphalia had the worst imaginable labor problems . . . . Local residents refused the indescribably dirty mill work. The company had to import its workers from the East and from the Ruhr district. It now found itself faced with a human conglomeration which was endlessly difficult to control . . . [and] reacted with boundless suspicion to any attempts to approach them. Finally,

the management . . . turned . . . to a woman trained in industrial social work . . .

A large rayon factory on the outskirts of a large north German city could not achieve stable worker relations . . . Naive country girls, solid working-class wives and far too experienced big-city girls produced a colorful, constantly changing mixture without internal cohesion. The factory council was without power or influence. . . . The management, stimulated by the propaganda of the recent period, experimented with industrial social work . . . . A somewhat older worker, educated in modern social thought, was hired as an industrial social worker. Following the Bielefeld method, she spent months [as a worker] and then approached management with a plan of action . . . aimed at awakening the active interest of the indifferent masses themselves in the plan.[52]

This model of industrial social work had originated at the Oetker firm in Bielefeld, where about 800 mostly juvenile women laborers were employed.[53] "Gefährdetenfürsorgerinnen" (social workers for those especially vulnerable), themselves all workers and members of free labor unions, worked at Oetker and a few other firms in the region, in order to "get to know their charges to the very depths of their beings." After several months these women were assigned to the intra-plant social work system. Considering their function as "non-political," they took pains to work closely with both the factory council and the union shop steward.[54] One failure of the Bielefeld system, later the cause of lengthy debates between employers and the DAF, was the fact that the social industrial workers were not direct salaried employees, but received from the employers only the normal factory workers' wages. The differential for a social worker's salary was paid by the "committee for Industrial Social Work," a body composed of the employers, social workers, and other "interested personages."[55] This arrangement was intended to insure the industrial social workers a greater independence from the employers.

The Bielefeld model of industrial social work emphasized not family welfare but social work applied to the factory work place.*

---

*A more precise translation of the term is "social industrial work": in the Nazi period it was changed to "industrial social work", reflecting a change of emphasis. The latter construction, more usual in English, is used in this translation for both periods.

The point of departure was the "differentness" of women, whose "sensitive nature" was repelled by the factory, a finding which is as old as women's factory labor:

> Factory labor oppresses a woman more and in a different way than a man. A woman's constitution is different; it is above all more sensitive. A woman can suffer horribly from things which hardly affect a man. This is a fact which is not to be taken lightly or smiled at. It would also be wrong to try to treat women the same as men. No, we must make it possible for the woman to develop and use her special abilities according to her situation, to obtain an influence over the economic process for her own and the general good. To this end, only women can help women.[56]

Dismantling these restraints of labor was the task of the industrial social workers. They were to begin immediately with the women's selection, work assignments, transfer, and termination.[57] The women's preferences were to be taken into account, with consideration given to whether a worker would

> rather work standing up or sitting, prefers a job where one can think or daydream now and then, or loves work at a rapid pace that carries her along so that the time flies: whether she would prefer to be in a specific work area, etc. All of these insignificant factors play a role with women.[58]

The goal of the Bielefeld workers was to make "intellectually, emotionally, and physically atrophied" workers and those employers who were alert to their suffering aware of the possibilities for "pleasure in work" and the means to a more sensible work process. The new organization of labor would reduce status differences and replace "external authority" with "inner mastery." To this end, the Bielefeld social workers' efforts concentrated on selecting supervisors and trainees primarily according to educational criteria—and only secondarily according to their technical abilities—and tried to introduce the foremen to more effective methods of social communications.[59] For, as one welfare worker noted:

> Women are particularly sensitive. Things that hardly affect a man will rankle a woman for days or weeks at a time. We

frequently have the task of counteracting sensitivity, or you
could say fussiness . . . The foreman usually has enormous
power, in a spinning mill, for example, through the assignment of machines or the allocation of materials of varying
quality. Those who are not in his good graces often have a
difficult time. A foreman who supervises 120 women said to
me that ''as a man, one can't always be fair. When Paula looks
at me that way I have to give her good yarn.'' Now, if a
woman worker is neglected, one can do something, especially
with an open-minded and sensible foreman . . . Another
worker displayed nervous stomach trouble. For four months
the doctor was unable to find anything wrong. The worker B.,
frequently had to interrupt her work. In a conversation with the
industrial social worker, it became apparent that B. felt an
insurmountable fear, actually terror, toward her foreman.
Ordinarily, one would try to talk to the foreman. But in this
case it was impossible, (the foreman was 60 years old, hard,
embittered, and taciturn) and since there was another worker
who was not bothered by the foreman's behavior who was
ready to exchange places, B. was transferred, and her stomach
problems ceased . . .

Other kinds of problems affected performance in the work
place, particularly when they became the subject of gossip;
such as a suspected abortion, dishonesty or the like. The
matter is completely out of one's control, but the gossip,
which so pleasantly fills a void in the workers' lives and is so
difficult to suppress, leads to needling, and the girl suffers.
The industrial social worker happens to hear about it, but
attempts to counteract the rumor are useless. Since the girl's
attitude and work are suffering, she is transferred.[60]

   The objectives of the Bielefeld social workers reflected the
guiding principles of the technocratic ''psycho-technology,'' or
labor science, which had emerged with the changing industrial work
process, itself a result of the continuing rationalization of labor from
the beginning of the twentieth century. Their job was to remove the
''emotional and physical limitations and sources of fatigue'' caused
by disruptive family life, poor communication in the workplace,
poor working conditions, or the work process itself. Their goal was
to heighten the women's ''pleasure in work'' or awaken it in the

first place. They presumed—particularly after the studies of this by Hendrik de Man at the Frankfurt Academy of Labor[61]—that the joy of labor had been lost but could be recovered, and that it was the key to extracting those final resources of productivity, which no amount of technical and organizational rationalization could reach. Industrial social work's aim was to tap this reserve by providing the "optimal psychological and physical arrangement of work," and thereby increasing profitability.[62]

The Bielefeld model did not, however, limit itself to the industrial work place; it also encroached on the workers' private lives. Labor and social theorists agreed that "the rhythm of piece work awakens a yearning for jazz; monotonous work the need for sensation." They openly confessed that "the mind-numbing lock step of the contemporary factory demands a counterbalance in intellectual and emotional life." But movie houses, dance halls, and coffee houses with jazz music, were not considered proper recreation for grown women and juveniles.[63] Instead, the Bielefeld social workers—much like the other industrial welfare workers—conducted home economics courses for laborers. But the Bielefeld model regarded these courses differently from previous social work systems. The courses were not just aids in creating a disciplined, domesticated work force, but were primarily "public educational work," designed to shake the "average woman worker" out of her "inner sluggishness," lethargic lack of initiative, and feelings of inferiority. Since women workers had a low level of participation in political parties and labor unions, the Bielefeld workers assumed that their intellectual interests were almost totally dormant, and that the way to first approach them was through courses of a practical nature, such as cooking, sewing, handicrafts, and gymnastics. Women who were too strongly inhibited to attend a union-organized event on their own initiative would participate in educational events led by persons they trusted, like the industrial social workers, and in familiar places, the factory. Once these courses were accepted by the women workers, they would be linked up with the union or the local adult education school.[64]

Before 1933, employers were not enthusiastic supporters of this model of factory-associated adult education: it had not spread beyond seven Westphalian companies. Employers distrusted the Bielefeld social workers' organizational ties to the free labor unions, an association that continued to be used against the industrial social work of the DAF Women's Bureaus during the period of National Socialism.[65]

The opinions of the Bielefeld social workers' trade union colleagues were varied. Some, like Gertrud Hanna, totally rejected industrial social work along with every employer-sponsored social policy, in favor of public welfare.[66] Others, like Eduard Heimann, liked the possibility of "educating the working class to solidarity and responsible organization of the work process," rather than completely "abandoning it to the opposition," meaning especially DINTA and its version of factory welfare:

> The problem is on the agenda. It will either be solved against the worker's movement and thus strengthen the attractiveness of the opposition or it will be solved with the active participation of the workers' movement furthering the interests of its ideal of a masterless and free discipline of labor, and thus be a powerful stimulus to the strength and optimism of the workers' movement.[67]

Women propagandists for industrial social work had no such second thoughts. They were confident of the imminent success of their endeavor: "[Industrial social work] might in one form or another be adopted by the state or the unions, but it will definitely be accepted by leading women workers."[68]

This confidence was soon justified. In 1933, just as the Nazis disbanded the trade unions, Ilse Ganzert, one of the innovators in industrial social work, contacted the new Reich Women's Leader and Director of the DAF Women's Bureau, Gertrud Scholtz-Klink, proposing the adoption of her model of industrial social work.[69] Several factors made her success possible: the DAF saw in the Bielefeld model, far more than in any of the others, a foundation for the development of an educational social work in line with the National Socialist *Weltanschauung*. This social work did not provide welfare, it trained people to help themselves.[70] The goal of the Bielefeld social workers' educational programs was eliminating female "apathy" and feelings of inferiority, substituting a personal interest and sense of responsibility in the labor process, the company, and the community.[71] The DAF's own goals were easily appended: promoting the "nobility of German labor," and a national socialist "labor ethic" pledged to the *Volksgemeinschaft* (national community).

Even more appealing was Bielefeld social work's emphasis on serving workers in the factory, and its only peripheral involvement in family welfare activities. This would help obviate organizational overlaps, and create a clear division of labor: factories, and the entire area of wage labor, were to be the exclusive social policy domain of the DAF; other institutions, such as the Nazional Sozialistische Volkswohlfahrt (National Socialist People's Welfare—NSV) and the NS Frauenschaft, were responsible for household and family life.

Another reason the DAF favored the Bielefeld model was its reliance on non-professionals for training industrial social workers. This employment of dilettantes, who were highly valued as long as they acted out of the correct "persuasion," was already the preferred prescription for National Socialist "reconstruction."[72] By transferring most of the training to the factory and, as far as possible, choosing candidates who had practical experience but no professional training—that is, either "leading workers" from the factory, the Reichsarbeitsdienst (Reich Labor Service), Bund Deutsche Mädel (League of German Girls, the BDM), group leaders, or nurses from the Nazi Party Welfare (NSV) organization—the DAF could bypass the educational monopoly held by the Women's Social Work Schools until 1933. The National Socialists had found the schools politically suspect and immediately after taking power, had suppressed or taken them over.[73]

The final and most persuasive reason for the DAF to adopt the Bielefeld model was its arrangement of the social workers' contractual relationship to the employer, i.e., the triangular contract between the employer, the "Committee for Industrial Social Work," and the industrial social workers. They had only to replace the Committee with the DAF itself to insure their influence on industrial social work and to limit the social workers' dependence on the employers in favor of direction by the DAF.

Thus a "Central Office for Industrial Social Work" was very quickly set up in the Women's Bureau of the DAF, led by Ganzert and Hanne.[74] In October 1934, this office organized a conference for plant social service workers and other interested parties at which the Reich Women's Leader, Gertrud Scholtz-Klink, announced the coordination and centralization of industrial social work. Her objectives were twofold: placing industrial social workers in all firms employing more than 250 women and prohibiting the employment of plant welfare officers who had been trained in Women's Social Work Schools.[75] Contractual provisions were arranged so that the industrial social workers were no longer hired by the employers, now called "factory leaders" (Betriebsführer), but by the Women's Bureau of the DAF, which would now have sole control over training, hiring, and firing of industrial social workers. The firms entered into a contract with the Women's Bureau and paid the social workers the usual wage for women workers plus an additional sum set by the Women's Bureau as an "efficiency" bonus. In the end the social industrial workers received roughly the same salary as the former welfare officer.[76] By the end of 1935, about forty industrial social workers were employed in accord with these provisions, and forty more were in the process of being trained by the DAF. At this point industry, which still employed about 380 factory welfare officers, began to offer resistance to the intrusion of the DAF into these intracompany matters.[77]

Chapter Four:
Petty Warfare
Between the Giants:
Industry vs. the DAF

The conflict between industry and the DAF was waged on two levels. The first was that of formal arrangements. The DAF wanted the greatest possible, formally guaranteed influence over industrial social work. The employers wanted to prevent the intrusion of any external authority not completely controlled by themselves. The battle was fought with a dogged tenacity and long-winded haggling over detail, swelling document files until the collapse of the Third Reich.

To combat the DAF's plan for the training and terms of employment of future industrial social workers, the business organizations involved—the Reich Economic Council, Reichsgruppe Industrie, and the larger industrial concerns already employing factory welfare officers—came to an understanding with one another and formulated a counter strategy. They quickly agreed that the three-party contract between the DAF, the individual firm, and the industrial social workers must not be allowed to become common practice. The factory leaders' exclusive social responsibility, embodied in the *Gesetz zur Ordnung der Nationalen Arbeit* (AOG) or Law for the Regulation of National Labor of 1934, was their most frequently used argument against DAF control. Industry immediately rejected the possibility of a DAF imposed "Social Commissar" in the person of the industrial social worker.[78] A later Director of the Reichsgruppe (a textile manufacturer, who was himself a supporter of the principle of industrial welfare) voiced his reservations: "If we ask employers to pay for something that someone else will control, we'll certainly find few takers."[79] Industrialists however, had nothing against additional practical training in the factory and the "development of a world view" in its industrial welfare workers, so long as this type of training was preceded by an orthodox social welfare education.[80]

The employers were able to get what they wanted in a formal agreement signed on 11 December 1935 between the heads of the Reich Economic Council, the Reichsgruppe Industrie, and the DAF Women's Bureau. The three-party contracts were dropped; the factory leaders would choose their social workers themselves (although the DAF could make suggestions), and salaries would be set and paid by the firm. The Reichsgruppe Industrie declared itself willing to use its influence to encourage a wider adoption of industrial social work. In return, the DAF insured its influence over training in the form of "monitoring the professional preparatory education and the ongoing orientation and instruction of women entering the field of industrial social work." Toward this end, all currently active plant welfare officers were to be summoned to courses "in ideological and pedagogical training." On successful completion of this training, i.e., emerging with the correct political orientation according to DAF standards, they would receive an "industrial social worker" certificate. Currently employed social workers could continue to work without this certificate, but beginning professionals were required to complete a factory internship directly in production, not in the industrial welfare apparatus.[81]

Despite this formal agreement, the DAF Women's Bureau was far from ready to concede defeat. The DAF continually tried to evade the provisions of the agreement, especially at regional and district levels, by reasserting their monopoly over selection and training, and trying to increase the social workers' obligation to the DAF.[82] At the beginning, the Reichsgruppe Industrie repeatedly issued denials of press descriptions of the industrial social workers as "DAF representatives." Later, the Reichsgruppe gave up, and this label was generally used.[83]

The DAF also demanded semi-annual activity reports from the industrial social workers, in order to obtain information about the disposition of problems in the women's industries. The Reichsgruppe Industrie was only able to modify this requirement by securing a proviso that, before being presented to the DAF shop steward for signature, the social workers' reports would first be shown to the factory leader.[84] Next, the DAF claimed exclusive authority over the placement of social industrial workers, but because of the objections of the Reichsgruppe Industrie the Reich Employment Office (Reichsanstalt für Arbeitsvermittlung) did not grant their demand.[85]

At the same time, the DAF increased its efforts to bring the social workers under political-ideological control by promoting the idea that industrial social workers should also assume the functions of supervisors of women workers. This meant the social workers would be direct representatives of the DAF, bound to its orders, and under greater control of the DAF shop steward. This "merging of the personnel" of both offices, industrial social worker and Betriebsfrauenwalterin (supervisors), became common but not universal practice. In 1944 there were still plant welfare officers who were not acknowledged as industrial social workers, and because of their refusal to participate in DAF training, these women were "ideologically suspect."[86] Therefore, in April 1944, the Director of the DAF, Robert Ley, wanted to combine both offices as a general rule, ostensibly because of "friction" between the DAF Betriebsfrauenwalterin and the social workers. In difficult cases the social worker would have to resign in favor of the DAF functionary, who was usually an ordinary worker. Employers who considered this measure completely unacceptable were able to substitute for its immediate enactment a gradual "merging of personnel." During this process, only women with a social welfare education would be allowed to exercise the double function.[87]

As Betriebsfrauenwalterin, the social worker now had the responsibility of forming women's groups in the factories. These were the feminine complement of the male plant groups which saw themselves as national socialist "shock troops of the DAF in the factories." A group consisted of at least six women workers or salaried employees, preferably aged twenty-five to thirty-five. After a three month "practice period," in which they were trained in "ability and attitude," they were certified as a plant women's group by the DAF regional Frauenwalterin.[88]

The activities of these "elite groups" of "the best women workers" were limited in practice mainly to supporting the welfare work of the social workers. However, they were, together with the male work groups, responsible for insuring the "worthy organization of leisure time" and for lending this time a "womanly accent." A "new work ethic" was to grow from these shared evenings of comradeship between "man and woman in the factory."[89] The DAF's larger plans for national and factory community "reconstruction," "training," and "orientation," were not limited to leisure time activities. The factory women's groups were supposed to be "the solid and reliable framework for the internal reconstruction of the female staff.'' Group members were to receive further training, as forewomen and apprentices, and would become the female "non-commissioned officer corps.'' Without them, female workers would remain "a disorderly mass, difficult to direct and hard to control, without morale or pleasure in labor.''[90] The DAF believed that this plan for the exercise of discipline over the female labor force by women from their own ranks was far better than an ideological "reorientation" of graduates of the Women's Social Work Schools through DAF courses.[91]

In many cases, the DAF succeeded in pushing through its preferred type of industrial social worker, especially in smaller and middle-sized firms with predominantly female labor forces. Up to 80 percent of these women were exposed to Betriebsfrauenwalterinnen, and thus to the direct influence of the DAF. This influence was so great that in several handicraft industries intercompany "social guilds" were organized in which industrial social workers were influential.[92] Small businessmen undoubtedly found it difficult to limit or control the influence of the DAF over these organizations. The large industrial groups, such as the Ruhr coal mines, IG Farben, and Siemens, had more success in warding off the influence of the DAF on industrial social work. Wherever possible, they preferred to hire "plant welfare officers" or "company social service workers" who had not been trained or indoctrinated by the DAF. This led to fresh sniping from the Women's Bureau of the DAF about the factory managers' too narrow understanding of "factory community" and their tenacious resistance to the "chain of command" in industrial social work as envisioned by the DAF.[93] The heavy industry employers avoided directly confronting the DAF's complaints. Their oft-cited position was that they employed only a relatively small number of women, or in the case of mining, hardly any at all. Thus the task of their social workers was family welfare, and the care of women workers in the factory work place (the central point of the DAF's "industrial social work") was at most secondary in their industrial welfare system. They flatly denied that the DAF had the political and social competence to exercise influence over the comprehensive family welfare systems practiced by the large industrial groups.[94]

The Ruhr district hard coal mining group was able to obtain a separate agreement with the DAF, according to which all plant welfare officers would receive "industrial social worker" identification cards, thereby gaining political security clearance without being investigated. Management, not the industrial social workers themselves, would submit the semi-annual activity reports to the DAF.[95]

In Siemens, which had employed "plant social service workers" since 1911 and in the 1930s had the largest female labor force in Germany, the DAF tried in vain to compel the employment of DAF trained social workers on a large scale. Not until 1938 would Siemens allow a DAF Frauenwalterin to be trained as a factory social worker, and then only one, in a cable factory.[96] Although Siemen's thirty social service workers occasionally took part in DAF training sessions, only two of them received or accepted DAF certification as "industrial social workers."

On the whole, Siemens largely succeeded in restricting the work of the DAF in its factories to the narrowest possible limits. This led to frequent complaints from the DAF district office. The DAF district steward for Siemensstadt said that

> he knew the firm especially the gentlemen from the social policy department, who with their Colgate masks and their "keep smiling" are always very polite, he got along fine with them, but they all knew what to think of one another. You could never get anything through.

He therefore tried to use direct conversations with plant social workers to gain some influence and obtain information about the social situation at Siemens. They proved to be "little Siemenses," however, which he attributed to the fact that their supervisor—the head of the women's section in the social policy department—was "a university woman," who "would attack with a hatpin if she could."[97] The centralized, unified form of personnel management which the Siemens social policy department strove for was a constant thorn in the side of the DAF, who viewed this form of social management as a violation of the immediate and personal relationship between "management and labor" as it had been postulated by the AOG of 1934.

The DAF's effort to counterbalance the Siemens social management system focused on the only industrial social worker in the entire firm who was bound to the DAF, the woman they had placed in the cable factory in 1938. The DAF wanted her promoted to "head industrial social worker," thereby assuring itself a greater influence over social management at Siemens. The firm's management refused to accept this scheme, citing the woman's lack of "necessary stature," "deficient training," and "inadequate" personality.[98] In a conflict that went on for years, in which even Reich Woman's Leader Scholtz-Klink intervened, Siemens outmaneuvered the DAF. They upgraded the staff member responsible for all industrial social work at the firm to "officer in charge of industrial social work and factory social services," instead of "head industrial social worker." An employee in that position no longer required the endorsement of the DAF.[99]

Chapter Five:
Factory or Family?
Industrial Social Work
versus Plant Family Welfare

In the last analysis, the wrangling between the DAF and the employers over spheres of influence in industrial social work was indecisive. The important questions were not the disputes over guidelines, competence, or who ultimately had decision-making power. The real issue, at least for women workers, was the divergent social and educational assumptions and goals. In her study, *Frauenarbeit im Dritten Reich* (*Women's Work in the Third Reich*, 1977) Dörte Winkler argues that the conflict was over who could present the best social service image to the workers, the DAF as a quasi-union, or the patriarchal, beneficent employer. Yet this thesis appears to leave out the most important question; namely, why did the employers or the DAF employ social workers in the factories at all? What did each of the contracting parties have in mind for women, including women factory workers and the wives and families of their workers? What was really at issue?[100]

The answer, surprisingly, appears to run counter to general assumptions about National Socialist "home and hearth" ideology. It was not the employers who, with great expectations, applied the new labor sciences and pedagogy to their female labor force. Rather, it was the DAF Women's Bureau which extolled the virtues of its industrial social workers as disciplined—and disciplining—labor educators. It wasn't the DAF that worried about the stability and the future of the German family, but the employers, who insisted on maintaining their own social service influence over the families of their labor force. The DAF wanted to replace the employers' influence with that of Nazi organizations, above all the Nationalsozialistische Volkswohlfahrt (National Socialist People's Welfare), but without doing the employers the favor of relieving them of their costs and burdens. In the end, it was their conflicting

views on the structure and function of the female labor force that led
to different approaches to factory, family, and labor market policy.

THE DAF PLAN FOR "INDUSTRIAL SOCIAL WORK"

In the course of the negotiations with the Reichsgruppe Industrie,
the Reich Women's Leader, Gertrud Scholtz-Klink, gave a talk on
15 May 1936 before the Social-Economic Committee of the Reichsgruppe Industrie: "To my dear German men."[101] Her lecture was
met with an embarrassing lack of interest among the invited representatives of industry: "It was shocking and disgraceful to discover
that, besides Mr. Counselor Cuntz, exactly two members of the
Committee took part. This crushing fact fortunately did not become
known to the two speakers [the other was the Deputy Reich Medical
leader, Dr. Bartels] as it was possible to fill the hall in time."[102] This
lecture is a rich source of information on the National Socialist vision
of industrial social work and contains the first plausible explanation
of why the DAF and the Women's Bureau struggled so uncompro-
misingly for influence over the industrial social workers and thus
over women.

Scholtz-Klink's talk began with a revelation that contradicted
official family ideology: "many German families, many marriages,
have been shaken, to put it mildly, by the National Socialist
ideology." She saw the cause of this in the refusal of wives to
follow their "little SA men" in their "revolutionary ideas" and
"unremitting onward drive." Many married couples were "growing apart." Of course, she did not want to call the negative attitude
of women necessarily "deliberate resistance"; it was rather the
result of "a gap in the education of women." Nevertheless,
women's behavior was threatening enough to justify a great campaign to reeducate the German woman "to spontaneous affirmation
of National Socialist demands." She saw an important role for
industrial social workers in this struggle.

The political indifference attributed to women since patriarchal
prehistory and applauded or deplored according to the current
political trend, was according to Scholtz-Klink no longer acceptable
to the National Socialists:

For us today it is unthinkable that women should be assessed
in the old style, that she is merely a chivalrously protected and

carefully tended being, who should best be confined at home in the kitchen and nursery, but otherwise not exposed to rough reality. . . .

We want to shape the woman who proves herself in struggle, who stands beside her man, who enters into a marriage with the resolve to be her husband's comrade and best companion in any situation. We want to have the kind of woman who reckons with the realities [of this] . . . life, who knows from the start the situation in which their nation finds itself, how her nation is getting along, what things are necessary to keep her people sound. . . .

The purpose (of this) is not to organize women as a counter-balance to men, as it was for the old women's movement, or to make them advocates of women's rights. Instead, the purpose of our women's organization is exclusively that of making the powers of woman in all areas of life useful to their entire nation, not by coercion, but by training the woman to make this a voluntary, proud, I would even like to say, queenly, gift to the people. . . .

We don't want the political woman in the old sense, fighting against men; we want no struggle of woman against man. Rather, we want cooperation between man and woman as equals. . . . We want woman who will stand beside man and respect her own limits.

Women were to be shown how to "accept of their own free will all of the things that their husbands see as necessary, and not only to accept them but to live them as well." In addition, as "independent beings" women were to become "the bearers of the responsible future of the German people."

Scholtz-Klink had women workers in mind. Their work was of two different kinds: they were obliged to serve the fatherland in the factory and in addition had to provide for a biologically superior new generation. This second assignment united them with "women of all social strata" throughout the nation. It was to be the task of the social industrial workers "to make the woman worker herself into an active collaborator and bearer of the collective interests of the German people" in each of her assignments. Similar goals had already been suggested, in a somewhat less elevated form, in the

Bielefeld social worker model for adult education. New, however, was the openly proclaimed idea that women should submit "voluntarily" and "compliantly" to male domination. This was then incongruously linked with the vague concept that men and women were "equal in rank"—an equality from which, however, women derived no rights, but only the additional duty of "making their strengths in all areas of life useful to their nation as a whole." New also was the application in practice of the racist hereditary theories which had been abroad for some time. Racial hygiene, "which neither the male Nazi Party cell leader nor other men [could] propose to the women," was supposed to be imparted to them by the female industrial social workers:

> You can have a lecture hall full of women of all stations; they listen and, with folded hands, say at the end: That is true, that is good, it is hard, but it is right, we understand that. But afterwards, gentlemen, comes the step of taking the mother by the hand and going with her and her child to the hospital and ultimately obliterating the life of this child by sterilizing it. No man can show a German woman how to do that. As a man you can stand next to her and say: You must do this, Mrs. Meier. Mrs. Meier nods her head and says: I understand that I must, Mr. Müller. But the last sacrifice, as it were, the proud, voluntary affirmation of this step can only be made clear to a woman by another woman. . . . What it is like, the feeling of having borne a child, you will never experience, only a woman can experience it. You can only stand by and be thankful. It is exactly the same—and this is a very serious thing—when you must take this life away again from a woman, when you must blot it out through a measure, which simply happens to be necessary.

"Orientating" plant welfare officers in racial hygiene was a matter of more than passing interest to Scholtz-Klink. It was a vital goal which the DAF Women's Bureau pursued in its conflict with the Ruhr coal mines. At the time of this speech, the National Socialists still had not been able to persuade plant welfare workers, most of whom were Catholics and graduates of the district Catholic Women's Social Work Schools. These women were not the "little emissaries" of the "Führer" that Scholtz-Klink wished for. On the contrary, she had the feeling:

that they strictly refused to say to their women that they gave their support to the Law for the Prevention of Hereditarily Diseased Children. And they refuse on these grounds: I am a devout Catholic and according to my religious convictions and what my priest has told me, that is a sin—please, gentlemen I can document these things—and since it is a sin, I will do everything I can to prevent these things being told to the women workers.

Clearly, continuing resistance to the implementation of the sterilization law (Law for the Prevention of Hereditarily Diseased Children of 14 July 1933) especially among the traditionally-educated plant welfare officers rooted in Catholicism, was a substantial motive for the DAF Women's Bureau's repeated attempts to supervise their work. The alternatives Scholtz-Klink offered the plant welfare officers were either reeducation as National Socialist eugenicists, "with the conscious pride of being a German woman," or the prospect of seeing their future careers blocked.[103]

But Scholtz-Klink's political power was not sufficient to carry this out, at least not against the large industrial concerns with traditions of plant welfare. Most of these companies stood behind their plant welfare officers—though not because of a critical attitude toward racial hygiene and eugenics (there is not a single word from employers in the entire body of relevant files) but out of other interests, which will be discussed below. Nevertheless, the Woman's Bureau did not succeed in forcing aside women for whom it had no guarantee "that they totally accept and affirm the Führer's measures" in "special fields of work" in the factory. It therefore preferred to separate the plant welfare officers and factory social service workers trained in the old way from the new industrial social workers by isolating each in its own professional group. This policy was adopted despite the Bureau's otherwise strong commitment to a unified "coordination" of organizational structure.[104]

As in other cases where its practical political power was not adequate, the DAF turned to indoctrination measures. Employers obligingly sent their social workers to DAF lectures as long as costs and lost work time did not weigh too heavily. The question of racial and population policy played a prominent part in the courses at the DAF training centers (one frequently-used center was located in Berlin's Wannsee district) to which the plant welfare officers and—

carefully separated from them—the officially-endorsed industrial
social workers were regularly summoned. The Reichsgruppe Industrie's response ranged from mere consent to active propagandistic
support.[105] The training in racial policy, under the general heading
"eugenic theory and racial research work," included "practical
application in work in the factory through explanations of hereditary
character and personnel management."[106] In another course students were required to give written answers to questions on
"Provisions for the Jewish Question." The Racial Policy Bureau of
the NSDAP gave them lectures on "Future Questions of Population
Policy," "Ancestral Heredity," and "Race and Art."

The participants were also urged to "pay special attention to
prolific families and [to] explain to the labor force the importance of
increasing the birthrate." Of course, they were to see to it that
children were not produced indiscriminately. Families with at least
four children were desirable, although illegitimate children were
problematic and "asocial large families" were not at all welcome.[107] In accordance with this population policy mission, the
industrial social workers were to give special emphasis to the care of
pregnant women in factories.

After racial hygiene and population policy, "people's health"
was the third great slogan which National Socialist social pedagogy
incorporated into industrial social work. The DAF, Nazi Party, and
Nazi People's Welfare all launched noisy campaigns for the
"enhancement" of the health of the people. In the forefront of this
program stood the broad reeducation of the German working-class
family to a healthy style of life. Hygiene was the key. At the
admonition of the industrial social worker, the German citizen and
his companion bathed or showered once a week; they used tiled
toilets provided with instructions for efficient and sanitary use.
Thanks to daily calisthenics they always had warm feet; and in case
of rain, they kept an extra pair of shoes and socks in their lockers in
the specially established dressing rooms. In addition, they regularly
ate a warm, vitamin-rich mid-day meal, prepared according to the
national food supply plan aimed at the most economical and productive utilization of foodstuffs. Sometimes more marmalade,
sometimes more fish, and, of course, *Eintopf* (soup or stew)
according to the direction currently pursued by the official consumption management plan.[108] That was, at any rate, the way it was
supposed to be. But changing the private habits and preferences of
the people was not an easy task. Hygiene reeducation began outside

the private home, in the workplace.[109] Hygienic facilities were installed in factories where women could be made accustomed to their use. But some urging was apparently necessary: "What is the use of lovely, bright lounges if the workers stay at their machines on their breaks to sleep or read novels?"[110]

Although the DAF Women's Bureau had charged industrial social workers with educating women workers in the hygiene, racial, and population goals of National Socialism, they were not granted the most important means of realizing this education program: they were not permitted to offer the independent courses on mothering and domestic economy which had been a favorite activity of the previous plant welfare officers. The Reich Women's Leader made this clear:

> As a basic principle we do not wish that very many firms carry out their own mothers' training classes, because we connect these mothers' training classes with the fraternization of women from all social strata. We declare that there is in fact only one common denominator by which all of the women of a nation can be brought together. That is their predestination as mothers. This is the same for all women; therefore, we do not want the maternity training classes separated into Labor Front courses, Women's Corps classes, Evangelical and Catholic classes; instead we want mothers' training classes for all mothers.[111]

In other words, what was at issue was who would get a grip on motherhood and the household: the "factory community" through its plant welfare officers, or the "National Socialist National community" through Party organizations like the NS Women's Corps, the Reich Mothers' Service and the NS People's Welfare. In the end, industrial social workers did provide courses on house-keeping, cooking, childcare, and sewing, because women workers and workers' wives withdrew from these offerings by the Party organization. As late as 1940, when the "system of indoctrination" had been in action for years, in contrast to women from the civil service and white collar strata, workers were significantly under-represented in mothers' training courses outside of the factories.[112]

To some extent, this may have been a result of the "heavy burden of labor," as the Reich Women's Leader declared: Perhaps, however, these women would have refused to be trained as "mothers of the people" even if they had been able to find the time. Whatever the causes of this failure, it led the DAF Women's Bureau to give up its opposition to industry-run courses on the factory grounds as conducted by industrial social workers.[113] It continued, however, to try to obtain entry to the industrial courses for the NS Women's Corps and to assert its goals in their content.[114]

The training in running a household, maternity and childcare, and practical housework that the industrial social workers offered came to be seen as part of the national programs for control of consumption, popular hygiene, eugenics, and increases in the birthrate. Just as for the Bielefeld social workers, training in housework was not seen as an end in itself, but as a vehicle for the "community oriented reeducation" of women and their integration into the national community. This attempt to commit women's housework and childbearing to the creation of a national community of genetically sound "community conscious" aryan Germans, constituted the National Socialist vision of industrial social work. As in so many other cases, this vision was not the Nazis' own creation, but something they had picked up and appropriated to the service of the racial and military goals of the regime.[115]

The application of their "motherly powers" to the rearing of a genetically sound new generation in an orderly, hygienic household was only one aspect of the "flawless performance" that was expected of "aryan" women workers.[116] In 1936 Scholtz-Klink asserted:

> In this reconstruction of our nation, which after all stands on an entirely different set of principles than before, everyone must participate, all must contribute their piece. We can no longer measure the German man's attitude toward the German woman according to the old rules which we might say, honored woman as a sex. For now that the Führer has granted women such a great share in his project, we must begin to honor woman as workers and expect this of men too. We must honor her work, not only as craft worker and producer, but also as a comrade sharing political responsibilities with the German man.[117]

Shortly thereafter, at the "World Congress for Leisure Time and Recreation" in Hamburg, a "factory leader" of the Reichsgruppe Industrie articulated the Party's expectations for women even more clearly than had the Reich Women's Leader:

Outside of our country one frequently hears the observation that the only ideal of the German woman is to stand before the stove, bear and raise children, and make a pleasant home for her husband. That is a little too narrowly construed. Our women and girls are just as lively as any others in the world. Nor can the economy do without their participation. They do understand their natural duties and they are happy to admit that their preferences lie in the same direction. They know how to unite work and family; they bear a noble sense of pride in their occupations and into their communities. . . .

For this reason it was important, "that not only working men, but also women involved in gainful employment learn to have pride of their occupations. The work of the industrial social worker is an example."[118]

Nonetheless, the "work and occupational pride" of the German woman did not yet appear to be very strong. Ilse Ganzert, the promoter of industrial social work to the DAF, declared in 1936 that: "[the women] are not yet all actively touched by these things called national community, factory community, service to others, service to the whole."[119] Even years later women still hadn't developed the necessary "seriousness" and had only a very "slight relationship" to their workplace and the factory community. This attitude became dangerous with the labor shortage during the war:[120]

Industrial social workers and their co-workers must try everything to awaken occupational seriousness and the desire to work, despite the fact that after marriage an occupation no longer plays the dominant role in a woman's life. The participation of women [in work] including married women, is a service to the Nation.

But it was not merely a question of getting women to "take up work" in the factories, with their "unchanging, soul-less motions," where their only interest might be in their pay slip.[121] The goal was an "active," "responsible," "mentally alert," and "enthusiastic" work comrade, in contrast to the "apathetic," "congenitally defective" women and girls, "who are in such sexual bondage to their husbands and friends that they lack the energy for any other involvement."[122] Even greater demands were placed on the industrial social worker who was supposed to accomplish all this. She was supposed to be "mature in experience," but "young, fresh, and cheerful" as well, full of "vitality," "motherly," and "diplomatic."[123]

Naturally, the DAF expected greater productivity from these newly-trained and expertly-supervised workers, even though they never used the psychotechnical vocabulary of the 1920s (terms like "enhancement of productivity" or "deprogramming anxiety") and never hinted at a direct connection between social education in the factory and high levels of production. Of course, now and then a social worker might arrange for changes in a department that had failed to meet production quotas because she had found a technical error or mistake in the organization of the work process. This sort of example was happily and frequently publicized in small news articles.[124] Less publicity was given the fact that this method could also be used to spot overworked and exhausted women, so-called loafers, or attempts at slowing production. After all, welfare workers were supposed to be stewards of trust, not inspectors. Other authorities, such as the labor office, the timekeeper, the foreman, women supervisors, and spies were there for the direct supervision and intensification of production.[125]

The social workers were only peripherally involved with the practical application and further development of "labor science," although the DAF would have preferred to have more influence for itself and its industrial social workers over the design of workplaces for women. As guardian of the national interest for population policy and public health in the factory, the DAF was concerned that "valuable woman power achieve the best productivity possible, while the woman is still protected for her future task of motherhood."[126]

But even within the DAF, other and in the end more influential offices than the Women's Bureau were responsible for the organization and physiology of women's labor.[127] The professed focal point of "industrial social work," as formulated by the DAF, was "labor pedagogy." This was not to be understood as occupational training, but rather as training in the correct attitude toward labor, that is, toward "German labor:"[128]

> We do not want to allow ourselves to become the servants of machines, but to try to make them serve us. We do not allow our humanity to perish at our work, but try to help it to new

power through a new work ethic. To that end, "industrial social work" is an ideal path!

Suggestions on how to realize this program remained vague. A constantly recurring idea was that the woman worker's "pleasure in labor" could be increased by eliminating her "personal inhibitions" in order to transform "hectic, unharmonious, spiritually oppressive work into orderly [labor], yielding satisfaction."[129] This was not always easy, however. The ideals of "pleasure in labor" of the Women's Bureau and its industrial social workers were not always cheerfully received by the women workers:

> A woman happened to have pretty patterns in the piles of her boxes. It was work on a production line. The industrial social worker said to her: "Doesn't it give you even a little pleasure?" She answered: "Gimme the time for pleasure!"[130]

The vaguer the goal, the more obscure the method, the more extensive was the catalog of tasks of the industrial social workers. They were supposed to "remove inhibitions" and "dissolve tensions" in the work force, participate in "hiring and firing," and "stimulate the [satisfactory] arrangement of the workplace." They were to influence "the attitudes of the employees" by mobilizing the "especially conscientious workers," organize factory staff events in line with "traditional German sociability," cooperate in the workers' council, and even be involved in the training of apprentices, which very rarely happened.[131]

The final important area of responsibility the DAF continually urged upon industrial social workers was "personnel management in the factory,"[132] whose long term goal was the "national socialist orientation" of workers. But this could only be reached through the gradual "reconstruction of work," eliminating the alienating character of factory labor. This knowledge alone was not much use. The DAF Women's Bureau could not control the technical structure of the work process in the factory and, for their part, the employers hardly gave the industrial social workers any chance to influence it. What remained then was to deal with "purely personal factors: a tyrannical foreman, spiteful co-worker," or the "attempt at heartfelt work on behalf of humanity in the factory."[133]

The tension between foremen and women workers was a problem that gained importance with the growing labor shortage and the increase of women conscripted into the factories during the war, especially women unused to factory work. During the war the DAF tried to see to it that women were trained as much as possible by other women, "who proved themselves better at it than the foremen first brought in to help."[134]

> A woman is better able to sympathize with the situation of the newcomer. She knows the initial problems and sources of error, and helps with patience and understanding to eliminate inhibitions about the machines and contact with the technical sphere in general. She also unselfishly passes on her experience and know-how. A man is always more reserved in this respect.[135]

Depending on the size of the factory and the number of women employed, either the industrial social workers themselves were supposed to take over the training or they were to supervise and coordinate the trainees. The DAF Women's Bureau set up special courses of instruction for this purpose. The social workers also supervised intra-industrial retraining courses and were involved in the selection of the participating workers.[136]

To sum up, the scheme for industrial social work advocated by the DAF Women's Bureau was tailored for women workers in the factories and applied only to the Germans and "aryans" among the labor force. Foreign workers and "non-aryans" were never mentioned. The families of the workers were given little consideration. The factory worker was to be "supervised," "trained," and "led" according to her assumed female characteristics: she was to be "oriented" to a work ethic dedicated to the "national community."

But the woman worker was also a bearer of children. Alongside or even before her "honor as a worker" stood her "honor as a sex." In return for this honor she owed the nation a high standard of racial purity and "congenital health" for herself and her children.[137] Training women workers in the consciousness of this dual "honor" was also the task of the industrial social workers. In the factories, they had direct responsibility for ensuring that the organization of work was compatible with women's reproductive role and "nature." In the area of family welfare, however, they were supposed to act as no more than intermediaries to the appropriate Party organization. But this division of social welfare responsibilities—to the Labor Front for factory work and the Party for housework—

could not be maintained in practice. For one thing, women workers withdrew from "Party" welfare, at least as far as it appeared to be just more work in the form of courses and training sessions; for another, the labor of women could not be divided among different administrative mechanisms, as we shall see below.

Chapter Six:
Plant Welfare
in Industrial Practice
Under National Socialism

The plant family welfare system, as it developed in the Weimar Republic, remained the primary and sometimes exclusive task of the social workers up until the first years of the war, at least in the large industrial complexes such as IG-Farben, Siemens, Ruhr Mining, and Ruhr Steel (Thyssen), despite the DAF's attempts to reorient its efforts. An author from the independent welfare service, who had observed industrial social work at major factories and who took pains to remain on good terms with the Reichsgruppe Industrie, reported as late as 1939, that "'the actual factory or plant welfare officer is by far the preponderant type (as opposed to the industrial social worker) and family welfare is the more important form of work.''[138]

FROM 1929-30 TO 1934-35

Between 1929 and 1935—the period from the world economic crisis through gradual economic revival—despite massive layoffs, the number of clients for the plant family welfare officers did not decline. According to the Siemens' welfare officers' annual report for 1930-31:

[In the] families which had been supported by several actively employed members in the previous, more prosperous years, there was now only a single breadwinner on part-time providing for several unemployable or unemployed family members. The average weekly income of families served by the factory welfare system was roughly 15RM—and seldom rose above 20RM for a family of four, five, or more. The cases of debt through arrears in rent payments increased at an alarming rate.

Increasing cases of undernourishment and child neglect were
again observed.

Company management was especially concerned that even workers
who had been with the company for years had had to go into debt
and become "in need of aid."

Although the number of applications for support was rising, the
sources of aid were diminished. For the welfare offices this meant
"more thorough counseling and support" in each individual case.
They distributed food and counseled housewives in domestic thrift,
which "frequently removed the necessity for larger assistance."[139]
But these means were hardly effective at counteracting the progres-
sive impoverishment of the workers' families caused by part-time
work or unemployment. Two years later reports showed "increased
demand on factory welfare officers for aid in cases of nervous
breakdown, not only of workers themselves but especially of those
housewives and mothers burdened with the cares of managing their
households."

The problem of family survival continued to stand in the
foreground as things gradually began to get better after 1934. The
plant welfare officers now gave special attention to the newly hired.
Many firms preferentially rehired old, proven workers whom they
had laid off during the crisis. The welfare officers advised these
workers, arranging support for the "reconstruction of their family
economy" and the "repayment to municipal welfare offices" which
now came due.[140]

FROM 1935-36 TO 1939-40

In the following years, until the outbreak of the war, the tasks set
for industrial social work were modified, first by the financial con-
solidation of the working class household, and second by the increasingly limited labor supply, itself the reason for the economic
improvement in the workers' income. Large concerns were once
again running profitably and paying comparatively high wages, and
it became possible to achieve, briefly, a goal which had eluded
welfare reformers since the end of the nineteenth century, when there
had been no long-term solution to the problem of mass poverty. This
goal was an "appreciable and welcome shift in welfare work from
financial support to a more advisory and coordinating role."[141] The

entire array of home economics courses for workers' wives and
married and adolescent workers fell into this category again, just as
in the 1920s.[142] In addition, social welfare work included "counseling and advising the entire staff and its dependents in all questions
of the conduct of life." The plant welfare officers mediated between
the workers' families and every imaginable public and private authority, including the landlords if the rent was not paid on time and
the grocers if too much had been charged.[143]

The second large domain of the plant welfare system was
industrial health policy. Here, the endeavors of the DAF to "elevate
the people's health" coincided with the interests of the factories
which, in the throes of the labor shortage, desired a low rate of
absenteeism and healthy, "productive" workers.

If the factory inspectors' reports of recorded achievements are
reliable, the DAF's campaign for the hygienic and sanitary outfit-
ting of the factories appears to have been a remarkable success.
Canteens, washing and shower rooms, exercise yards, parks, and
occasionally even swimming pools sprang up.[144] Monitoring of the
hygiene of these facilities was the responsibility of the plant welfare
officers. At the same time it was they who—as the DAF had
directed social industrial workers—encouraged health and hygienic
measures for the women workers, organized "sport and gymnastic
classes," and set up and supervised the "schedule" for the use of
the factory bathing facilities.[145]

The largest and perhaps most important part of their work in the
field of health care, however, consisted of promoting a "healthy"
and "hygienic" standard of life in the workers' own households.
This often began as an attempt to stop the spread of disease, particularly tuberculosis, which was carefully monitored in factories in
the 1930s. Preventive measures included examinations in the plant's
own lung-care station, and home visits by the plant welfare officers,
who afterward procured sufficient beds if each family member did
not already have his own, and sometimes arranged for a comprehensive "reorganization of the apartment." Of course, the housewife
would here again be counseled in nutrition and economy.[146]

The employer's goal of course, was to reduce absenteeism. The
social worker's judgment, experience, and position of trust with the
worker's family could aid in determining the seriousness of so
subjective a condition as illness.[147] However, the "factory community" was not always characterized by a "relationship of trust."
With a growing labor shortage and increasing worker mobility,

"asocial" workers often came under the surveillance of the plant welfare system. The threat of dismissal no longer had a disciplinary effect, and sickly, work-shy, or unstable workers from "big-city families" could not be exchanged for "healthy" and "efficient" ones from "respectable" households. A greater portion of industrial social welfare was now aimed at "illness and pregnancy care" which, depending on the firms' internal classification of clients, could turn into strict monitoring of illness:

> The point of departure here is the daily contact of the I.S.W. with all of her fellow workers. There is also a weekly discussion of the week's sick list, in which all department heads participate as well. In every instance they determine: (1) whether assistance should be given in the case of long-term illness . . . (2) whether it is a matter of a good and diligent co-worker or if a case of work-shyness is suspected. In the latter case the illness will be strictly monitored; (3) whether a sick or family visit should be made by the I.S.W. or the department head. As a rule, in cases of serious illness, good long-term employees are given assistance to bridge the waiting period until health insurance payments begin.[148]

The care of the "long-term workforce" or the "strict supervision" of the high-turnover workers of "asocial" origins went beyond the immediate issues of illness and absenteeism and aimed at a longer-term workforce policy. Many employers were of the opinion that a true plant welfare system would only "pay off" after "longer periods of time," that is, "in generations," and then only in the case of plants located in rural regions with a comparatively stable laboring population.[149] That the employers in the provinces really did think in terms of generations and acted accordingly is demonstrated by the following example of plant welfare work in a paper factory in Baden:

> A character card is maintained for each child [of a staff member], in order to maintain a running record and in the interests of the firm, since our work force is local and stable and tends to be recruited largely from the children of our own people. These cards are also a record for the hiring of apprentices in the factory.[150]

But it was not only employers in remote rural regions who practiced generational care of their labor force. Siemens, too, kept internal records of families whose members had worked for the firm for several generations, and gave preference in hiring to their off-spring.[151] The "generational care" in the form of welfare, moni-toring, and selection of future workers according to criteria of their industrial suitability began almost before birth. Many firms provided remuneration to pregnant workers. Long-term workers received ad-ditional support during their maternity leaves, while others had to get by with sick pay, less than regular wages, and the usual package of diapers.[152] Whether this practice was prevalant or whether the claim made in 1939 by the Reich Women's leadership is true—that at the urging of the Women's Bureau 80 percent of factories made up the difference between regular pay and maternity benefits—cannot be determined from the available sources.[153] In any case, it appears that the occupational safety rules for pregnant women and the protection of mothers were more seriously heeded during the years before the war. With the organization of the DAF, workers managed to compel respect for maternity protection provisions as the employers' tribute to Nazi national biology. This was so that employed mothers, too, could "achieve their greatest contribution to the national community, by bearing healthy children despite difficult living conditions."[154] This intra-factory pregnancy and maternity care was supplemented by home visits to women workers as well as workers' wives. The plant welfare officer rarely came "empty handed," but in addition to the obligatory package of diapers, brought "a bottle of wine, apple juice, candy or the like."[155]

The increasing significance of maternal protection was, however, not merely the result of DAF Women's Bureau policy, the National Socialist population policy, or the propaganda circus over mother-hood. It stemmed, rather, from the very opposite of what National Socialist propaganda on motherhood proclaimed; specifically from the fact that there were more and more employed mothers in the factories. According to Siemens' records, the plant welfare system experienced "growing difficulty in placing the children in day care centers or nurseries. [During the] orientation of new female workers "the advising of women on their own households and children concerning time-planning" took on a special significance.[156]

Up to the beginning of the war, the family welfare model developed and applied in the factories before 1933 continued to be the focal point of industrial social work:

> If a firm employs men exclusively or predominantly, the assistants of the firm leaders will have to orient their work

primarily toward family welfare. If, on the other hand, the work force is primarily or mostly women, then counseling in the work of the workplace becomes the core of welfare work. If, however, among these women are mothers of families, then here again, and here especially, family welfare steps into the foreground.[157]

In fact, however, the family was almost always the center of interest for factory welfare activity, even when it was directed at young, unmarried, and childless women workers—as the previously cited example of the Oetker firm suggests:

> It is apparently an unwritten law of the working staff, that a young woman worker remains in the plant until her marriage. She belongs to a great plant community, the so-called "clearheaded family." She puts all of her strength in the service of the community and she receives from it not only her livelihood, but also protection and care in all life situations, counseling and aid for herself and her family members, health care, continuing education and domestic training, and finally a substantial grant for acquiring a trousseau.[158]

If any kind of welfare work directed at labor education was practiced at this time, it was of secondary importance, and was chiefly for workers who did not need family welfare, those who "did not live with their own families and thus lacked the protection and care of a domestic community," among whom "a relatively high level of turnover predominated," and who came "from the so-called asocial families of the metropolis." But welfare workers tried to give even these workers "encouragement and guidance to more pleasant and profitable leisure time activities;" through "cooking classes and maternity classes" or, for example, a "let's discover embroidery" contest organized by the factory newspaper and the factory women's group.[159]

FROM 1940-41 TO 1944-45

During the war, the problems confronted by industrial social work did in fact lean more heavily toward the labor-education end of the system. Conscripted German women and foreign female forced laborers became the social workers' newest and most problematic target group. From the beginning of the war, "the work of the factory social service worker [at Siemens] was significantly influenced by the increasing engagement of foreigners. By April 1945, over thirty welfare officers were employed at Siemens."[160] However, the records contain only a few references to the social workers' duties toward the foreigners, and exact descriptions of tasks and activities are lacking. One learns only that the social workers were responsible for "lodging" the foreign women, for the "establishment and surveillance" of their camps, and in the case of "Eastern workers" for coordinating "camp leaders" trained by the DAF or by the firms themselves.[161] That such activities were covered by the term "care" is not surprising since the distinction between supervision and control was already very fine as it applied to the less "productive," or "work-shy" German workers.

The lack of information can perhaps be explained as the result of the lack of concern about the social-pedagogical treatment of foreign laborers; in their case it was not necessary for Germans to renounce the direct application of force or even try to conceal it. The conscripted German women, however, were a different matter. According to the claims of the DAF, they were "under the special protection" of the industrial social workers, and as far as possible were to be placed only in work positions which the social workers had already tried out themselves, in order to be able to assign the workers "appropriately according to health, age, and ability."[162] Whatever else their "special care" may have included, the conscripted German women became the group most discussed in connection with industrial social work. What mattered to the social workers was "that the frequently reluctant conscriptee inwardly confirmed the necessity of her assignment and took a positive attitude toward her new, though often uncomfortable, work. She must be helped over the difficult period of acclimatization with great sympathy. Upon the new girl's first impressions depend not only her own enthusiasm for work and her productivity, but possibly the morale of an entire department."[163]

The DAF's labor-pedagogical program hoped to eliminate the problems of conscripted labor by encouraging women to volunteer for labor service; those very women who had not been ready to volunteer for drudgery in the munitions plants and had not been forced into the factories by economic duress. Predictably, the

program failed. Voluntary registration for the wartime labor force
was practically non-existent.

As early as 1940, the Reich Women's Leader had pointed to "an
embarrassing result" of the previous advertising campaigns for the
labor mobilization of women:

> For employment we only get those who know what work is.
> We also get the so-called upper ten thousand, above all
> officers' wives and people whose sense of honor can be
> captured. We absolutely cannot get certain upper-middle-class
> women who were not that well off before, who didn't learn all
> that much but who married well and now sit on their good
> bourgeois prosperity and pretend to be deaf at every call to
> even the easiest employment. They are people who live
> according to the old egoistic principle: Now that we have made
> it, now we will first look after ourselves; in a couple of years
> we can have ourselves a child and then perhaps another one.
> It's all figured out how it fits best. The kitchen cabinet comes
> with the second child and the radio or dressing room mirror
> with the third child. These people are hard to win to a selfless
> idea or one that is useful to the community.[164]

The DAF's "Institute of Labor Science," closer to industrial
practice than the Reich Women's Leadership, also put the problem
of women's inadequate motivation to work into material terms:

> The woman does not [find] her way to a specific activity from
> a personal interest in the practice of a certain occupation or
> from the goal and meaning of the task itself. Instead, the
> woman lets herself be led primarily from the perspective of the
> material return for her activity.[165]

The industry-supported Reich Board of Trustees for Efficiency
(Reichskuratorium für Wirtschaftlichkeit) offered a similar analysis
of the problem:

> When a woman comes into the world of work, to which she
> has yet no inner relationship, she is first confronted with and
> alienated by the excited and pompous behavior of the men.
> She is overcome by the multitude of impressions and facilities.
> Lack of understanding, however, calls forth indifference and

apathy. The money must in some way make up for all of these unaccustomed things, the extra load at home, the worry about child care, the poorer management of the household.

All of this leads to this result: when women being hired are asked what kind of work they would like to do, most explain: It's all the same to me what I do, the main thing is that I can earn something.[166]

There was not, in fact, much to be earned. For one thing, a portion of the wages of military wives was deducted from their husbands' allotments. For another, the wage freeze allowed hardly any raises. Finally, even when higher wages were gained there was little they could buy, since all essential commodities were rationed. The result was that the discipline of both conscripted and volunteer women workers was a constant cause for complaint:

The reasons for the inadequate labor discipline are essentially the following: Favorable financial situation and high level of support ("you no longer need to work"); lack of insight—the idea of the great goal of the war and the war community is foreign to most women; reluctance to work on the part of women employed as a result of the labor registration decrees; and the bad example that they set for the other women who were already working. Even conscripted women would work better if they didn't see shirkers on all sides.[167]

Conscripted women were, to put it in the military jargon which predominated in the debates over the deployment of female labor, a "real herd of sows"; an "undisciplined," "unstructured mass." Lacking even the slightest "interest in work," they frequently called in sick for unverifiable reasons and even went so far as to get pregnant. They "stirred up" one another, rattled the supervisors and foremen and undermined morale in the factory.

These problems became increasingly critical during the course of the war, as more and more women who had never worked in a factory before were conscripted. In these circumstances, industry became more willing to give labor education a chance, just as the DAF had demanded from the beginning. After 1942, even at Siemens for example, employers could think of no other solution than shifting from their earlier, chiefly family welfare-oriented social work to a heavier emphasis on "care for the working woman in the workplace." The plant social service workers henceforth took part in training newly-hired women, and they were consulted in cases of internal transfers. They were "brought into discussions between foremen and plant engineers" and more intensely trained in "electro-technical work processes."[168]

Other firms attempted to show the women good examples of German readiness for sacrifice. As the National Women's Service had already done in the First World War and as Marie-Elisabeth Lüders had recommended in 1936 on the basis of her previous experience with the War Office in that war, this effort was buttressed by the cooperation of students, academics, and other women working as volunteers, who were organized into "Volunteer Work Brigades." Reports of their success, such as the following, should, however, be taken with a grain of salt: "The enthusiastic, selfless, punctual engagement of these women had a splendid effect on the other women who now ceased their irregular work habits and became conscious of their duty."[169] Other reports acknowledged that even the wives of the "political leaders" (Nazi party officials) and of civil servants could "only with difficulty be won to honorary service" in positions such as "factory replacement, harvest, or neighborhood aid." In an effort to promote volunteerism, the NS Women's Corps drew up lists of women who were "expected to maintain an especially exemplary standard of behavior because of their husbands' positions" as factory leaders or salaried staff in private business. These were turned over to the district leader of the Labor Office.[170] Presumably, a volunteerism elicited in this coercive fashion could not have raised work morale in the factories to any degree. It was in fact more likely to have created new clients for the social workers.

The Labor Allocation Administration, looking for further ways of bringing women into the factories and maintaining their productivity, hit upon the idea of part-time work, for which they expected voluntary registration. The Labor Office called upon companies, "despite the industrial difficulties involved, to prepare themselves to introduce part-time employment for some women."[171] This plan, however, also failed; there was still not an adequate number of volunteers. Those part-time women who did sign up undermined the morale of permanent and full-time female employees to such an extent that the social workers racked their brains to find ways of organizing the workshops and the work flow to avoid conflict. Thus, for example, it was suggested that the women work only three days a week or be assigned to work every other week. Many firms went so far as to set up special workshops for part-time women to isolate them from the others. Social workers also tried to persuade the part-timers to work full-time.

The firms, on their part, were not interested in half-time work. They even accused the press of having presented far too rosy a picture of women's work and above all of having oversold the idea of half-time work. Whenever their personnel needs allowed, they refused to hire half-time workers. They did not want to involve themselves in costly technical readjustments in production methods, since the labor shortage was believed to be a temporary problem which could be solved more efficiently with full-time conscripted or foreign labor. Industry therefore resisted with every means at hand the expansion of the half-time work promoted by the DAF, with its possible negative effects on morale, service mindedness, and the deep-seated bias in favor of "German labor."

Women workers used the friction between the Labor Adminis-tration and the employers to their own advantage and "gladly played Labor Bureau and factory against one another." "In practice the situation of the Labor Bureau is often this: factory management requests the assignment of women, indicating that X-number of half-time workers are also needed. When the women report to the lower administrative department it turns out that there is no half-time employment available." Thus women assigned by the Labor Office to half-time work could expect to be rejected by the factories.

Naturally, women portrayed the state of their health to be as poor as possible in order to remain exempt from conscription, or at least to be classified as half-time workers. The Labor Bureaus, however, quickly reacted "with stricter measures" and assigned almost all unemployed women to industrial work. When some of them collapsed physically after a few days it became the task of the social workers to separate the malingerers from those women who were truly overworked and totally exhausted, to isolate women who resisted coercion from those who were resigned or unassertive, and to guarantee a minimum of labor discipline.[172] This was a gargan-tuan labor-pedagogical effort and it is very doubtful that they succeeded. The secret "Reports from the Reich," prepared by the SS Security Service (Sicherheitsdienst or SD), frequently under-scored women's "loafing," "shirking," and "refusal to work," especially after the issue of the "Regulation for the Registration of

Men and Women for Assignment in the Defense of the Reich'' in January 1943.[173]

This failure in industrial integration of women probably explains the renewed campaign in 1944 by the DAF Leader, Robert Ley, which aimed at replacing plant welfare officers who had not been approved by the DAF with the more ideologically-fit factory Frauenwalterinnen. These non-DAF officers had been indirectly accused by Ley of being responsible for the women workers' lack of discipline and, thus, for the failure of the labor education concept. Industrial employers' protested because they believed that they simply could not afford to abandon factory welfare. This was despite the fact that by this time productivity and increased efficiency were the blatant aim of all factory policy, undisguised by pretensions to national or factory community. The newly-conscripted women were, for the most part, married, and in addition to their housework frequently had children to care for. During the war, the proportion of such women workers had increased,[174] and this led to a greatly enlarged family welfare agenda for the industrial social workers.

These workers' primary concern, however—the care of children—had long since been taken away from the factories by the National Socialist People's Welfare Organization. The latter had managed to take control of the recently organized factory crèches and kindergartens over the opposition of the firms, which continued to the very end of the war.[175] The NS Women's Corps had also concerned itself with the placement of the children of employed women, in part by organizing ''neighborhood support groups.'' Between these support groups and the 1.2 million kindergarten places available during the war, child care was relatively well-handled. Plant welfare officers had to intervene and mediate in this area only in special cases.[176]

Another problem, less easily resolved, was the claim of husbands over the labor power of their wives. In certain circumstances the husband, if the so-called Guardianship Court had granted his petition for authority, could assert *his* right to *his* wife's termination of employment without notice. The prerequisite for such a step was ''that the employment of his wife was damaging to the marital interests.'' For, ''in general, it is self-evident that in a question of infringement upon marital interests, questions of employment must assume secondary importance.''[177]

Everything wasn't on the husband's side, however; in wartime they had to expect "inconveniences" and, as one jurist put it: "In principle, the State has already insured that grave infringement of marital interests shall not occur".[178]

Those affected husbands, especially soldiers at the front, saw matters differently, and bombarded the Labor Bureaus with "rude letters" in which they expressed such sentiments as, "their wives should not have to work, because they are on the battlefield, after all, and that should be enough."[179] "If the Fatherland's reward to its soldiers is supposed to be that after risking his life he comes home to find a sick and worn out wife with whom to finish out his life, it is an astounding reward."[180] In response to such attitudes social workers in general "all concurred in complaining that husbands did not show sufficient appreciation of the duties resulting from the employment of their wives . . . [and] propaganda was urgently needed to influence the men."[181]

Although the High Command of the Wehrmacht circulated letters and "Communiques to the Troops" using their greater appreciation of the problems of working wives, in the final analysis it fell to the plant welfare officers to support the Front, see to it that despite factory work households were kept in some kind of order and, in addition to all of this, to bring about a reduction in women's absenteeism.

> Since the beginning of the war, the amount of women's lost time has increased by leaps and bounds due to the extensive special leaves and legitimate absences caused by necessary trips to the authorities, wash days, errands of all descriptions—reasons which are associated with the war and in which Berlin as a metropolis plays a special role.[182]

Thus the plant welfare officers were especially concerned with working women's management of time. They encouraged appropriate planning by granting and assigning housework days, which were naturally unpaid, to be claimed in certain circumstances. Welfare workers also took over certain household tasks, which during the course of the war led to a partial cooperation with the National Socialist organizations, as had happened with labor-pedagogical social work. They began "mending-basket actions" in which the working women's torn linen was collected and repaired by women in the Reich Women's Corps, Reich Labor Service or BDM groups. Since shopping in particular had become more nerve-wracking and

time-consuming, industrial social workers organized shopping services and set up sales outlets in the factories.[183]

The marital interests that could be asserted by the husbands of
conscripted workers were not limited to insistence upon a well-run
household. There was also a matter of avoiding emotional "disrup-
tion" and sexual "alienation." Thus, the industrial social workers
often had to mediate between women workers and management
regarding special leaves. Such leave could and was supposed to be
granted on short notice when husbands or fiances came home on
leave from the front. It was subtracted from normal vacation time;
if this was already used up, additional leave could be granted which,
of course, was unpaid, as were the housework and wash days. If the
firm felt it could not dispense with the worker's labor, the industrial
social worker could try requesting a woman "factory replacement"
from the NS Women's Corps, who would work without pay. NS
Women's Corps' interest in these special leaves was outlined in their
magazine "NS-Frauenwarte":

> At this time we are frequently seeing women whose husbands
> have been away in the armed services for some time, coming
> to doctors with complaints of infertility. They then report that
> they have already been married for a number of years, that the
> husband is, of course, a soldier, but had already been home on
> short leave once or several times. Certainly, many a woman
> has the good fortune that her husband's short leave is fruitful
> in this, the truest sense of the word, but on the other hand, we
> must keep in mind what has just said about development and
> acclimatization in marriage. Directly between two periods,
> that is between the tenth and eighteenth days, the best
> possibilities for conception occur. Not infrequently we observe
> that separation of the marital partners at just this time can be
> a cause of infertility. The importance of just these consider-
> ations for wartime leave need only be noted in passing.[184]

Despite housework days, special leave granted by the firms, and
doubtful advice on the part of NS women's publications, marital
problems remained on the agenda until the end of the war. In these
circumstances employers felt responsible for doing whatever they
could, through their various social workers. The latter exerted
themselves mightily in the interests of the families of drafted
soldiers and women workers, so that "no damage should occur,

especially to the raising of the children, as a result of the war.''[185] Social workers organized Christmas presents for the children and occupied women workers' and workers' wives' scant leisure time in knitting stockings for their drafted ''work comrades,'' and producing squares for the NS People's Welfare's wool blankets. All of this, accompanied by ''song and conversation,'' was to instill in them a ''sense of sacrifice'' and ''community spirit.''[186]

During their monthly home visits the social workers personally distributed the supplementary family support paid by the firm, thus making clear the source of the funds, namely the company and not public welfare. Employers wanted to keep their workers' families and the wives of drafted workers as far removed as possible from public support, since in their eyes state aid during a ''temporary emergency,'' was equated with ''demoralization,'' a condition from which those affected might not be able to escape on their own.[187]

Chapter Seven:
Conclusion

This study has shown that industrial social work, far from being an empty gesture at public assistance, was in fact the embodiment of attitudes deeply embedded in social and political interests and strategies. For one segment of entrepreneurs, especially those of the Ruhr industries, industrial social work, with its origins in the numerous industrial policies of the nineteenth century, was an established part of business. For another group, the electric and chemical sector, industrial social work was an integral factor in the process of comprehensive rationalization and fundamental reform of industrial policy in the 'twenties. The National Socialist organizations, especially the DAF and its Women's Bureau, regarded industrial welfare work as a means of indoctrinating women workers in their racial, labor and political programs, thereby increasing the profitability of the female work force.

The discussions between industry and the DAF concerned the political aspect of industrial social work as much as the control of its content and methods. These exchanges demonstrate once again that National Socialism was no monolithic system, no homogeneous dictatorship responsible for everything that occurred in industry. Clearly, the employers maintained a considerable amount of discretion, which they believed necessary to achieve their own social and domestic political goals. Although they vehemently and effectively rejected many encroachments on their industrial and family policies, employers saw no reason to oppose the attempts by the DAF to indoctrinate industrial social workers in its racial and political ideology.[188] In its turn, the DAF policy of pedagogic conditioning of working women ran counter to the National Socialists' typical attempt to restore women to the home.

During the period of the world economic crisis and continuing through the gradual recovery from mass unemployment up to the later 1930s, family welfare was a form of crisis management for the worker household, the continued existence of which, even on a minimal level, required continual safeguarding. These efforts achieved a certain success, as workers' incomes began to rise again. The following period, through the early war years, was characterized by an increasing shortage of labor. For working families, this meant a higher income, due less to wage increases than to the fact that shifts were lengthened and more family members were employed. In these circumstances a worker could afford to stay in bed when sick, switch workplaces, or even risk missing a day to recover from a hangover. From industry's and government's points of view, this freedom had to be checked. In addition to the industrial discipline apparatus already in place, a system of industrial family welfare was needed which would monitor private standards of living, in particular hygiene and health.

From now on, all women in the industrial workforce, whether they were already established workers or had been conscripted or were the wives of employed or retired men, mattered to industrial welfare in the family domain. This welfare work was more strongly pursued the more the maintenance of family relations was jeopardized by the influences of the war—by men's military service, bomb damage, evacuations, billeting of soldiers, rationing.

Industry's intentions in the industrial welfare programs can easily be seen in contemporary developments. Employers' interests demanded a family living arrangement in individual private households for its workers. Here in the home, in spite of women's gainful employment, a cheap but continually useful, orderly, healthy, neat, and disciplined labor force would be maintained, which would feel itself committed to both family and industry. Toward this end, employers established a system of control and disciplinary methods and engaged social workers, "housewives of industry" with a "motherly" capacity for sympathy, to act as mediators between employees and industrial management. The social workers might consult with the work force, try to attract them with some form of aid and, with gentle pressure, obtain influence where the traditional intra-industrial disciplinary system could hardly reach: the household domain of the workers and their dependents.

At the same time, because of its need for more and more women factory workers, industry combined unpaid housework and paid factory work into modern "dual work," which became less and less economically avoidable for the women of the proletariat. Wage policy was an important factor in the implementation of this system. The wage had to be high enough and variable enough to serve as a discipline and reward system, and it had to remain below the standard which might make it possible for women to maintain an acceptable independent existence. Analogous to this, men's wages had to be so designed that supplementary work by the wives was necessary or highly desirable.[189] Monotonous, repetitive piecework was assigned to women primarily as a justification for their lower wages, but also because there was little danger that such work would turn the women too far away from their "family cares and joys." Conversely, women presumably could withstand the monotony of this type of work, the kind that one would not ask a "German man" to do, precisely because they had a spiritually stimulating and physically relaxing balance in the realm of housework and childrearing.[190] If now and then the compulsion toward this dual work should not prove strong enough, then it became the responsibility of the welfare worker to convince the women that the drudgery of the factory was to be borne for the benefit of their children; that they were earning money not for themselves, but for their families.

INDUSTRIAL SOCIAL WORK AS PART OF THE NATIONAL SOCIALIST WOMEN'S POLICY

Among various elements of the National Socialists, women's policy diverged widely: the "old warriors" from the National Socialist Women's Organization combined the picture of the "German comrade" with ambitious career dreams of their own; the unemployed men of the SA and NSBO wanted to drive women back to home and hearth in order to assume their places as wage earners; and the DAF, seeking to aggrandize its organization, tried to establish itself up as "guardian" of national biology and employed women. Even in peacetime the NSV was beginning to prepare the community for future support of the war effort, and armament technocrats were planning a double burden for women analogous to that which already existed in industry.[191] Finally, the wartime labor market demanded the "total" employment of all women.[192]

Even in wartime, National Socialist women's policy pursued varying and often contradictory goals. Just as the campaign against double wage earners from 1924 to 1934–35 had frequently exempted both highly qualified women and those in the lowest-paid, "women's positions," many women were now recruited for the factories, while others could only maintain their marriage loans by giving up their jobs. Meanwhile, "selective breeding" was encouraged by tightening up the ban on abortion and by forbidding sex education and the sale of contraceptives; conversely, "selection" and "elimination" were furthered by the laws on sterilization and race. Women—as if not already burdened enough with all this— were also called upon to perform all kinds of "voluntary service."[193]

Although actual practice continued to be inconsistent, the creation of a "voluntary emergency service of the German woman" extricated the Nazis from an ideological dilemma, while providing a means of controlling all women and exploiting the female labor force. This instrument was effective because of the atmosphere of state terrorism. The pivotal point of National Socialist women's policy became the conditioning of women for conscription.

But the National Socialist plan for a comprehensive system of conscription of women for the "nation" was both politically and economically unsound. The women who performed their service in the factory proudly and willingly often did so in the belief that a woman who carried out her service to the community and fulfilled her obligation to the fatherland as a man did could also claim the same rights as a man. For other women who had quite enough work, both regular and supplementary, their position as wives and mothers in the national community (happily mistaken for egalitarian) served as a convenient argument in the resistance to factory work or any other unreasonable demand. Other workers resisted being removed from the home to work for "victory" and the good of "the fatherland and the community" not only because the factory was detrimental to their children or evoked the displeasure of their husbands, but because they feared persecution if not enough work could be exacted from them.

DIVERGENCE BETWEEN EMPLOYERS' AND NATIONAL SOCIALIST WOMEN'S POLICY

Where in fact were the battle lines drawn between the employers and the National Socialists? Where did the breach lie between entrepreneurial and National Socialist goals for the women's labor force?

During the period before the war these conflicts were open. The entrepreneur employing women had to reject or try to minimize everything that might decrease the availability of the female work force aged twenty to thirty. The early National Socialist "Home and Hearth" ideology was a definite infringement on this work potential. Political provisions concerning race and population also threatened to become intrusive, since employers wanted dual work adapted to conditions dictated by the needs of industrial production. National Socialist social policy, which would lead to more marriages and children for women workers, only increased the necessity for employers, whether they agreed with the policy or not, to prepare industry for a broadened range of dual work. Although their wage and social policies were deemed useful as industrial/political instruments, the National Socialists' labor education policy was considered to be superficial rhetoric.

For instance, industry considered it inappropriate to adopt women's health protective measures to the extent prescribed by groups outside of management, such as the DAF, the Women's Bureau, or the industrial social workers. The women of the DAF, for their part, did not trust management to provide a suitable level of consideration and indoctrination for women factory workers as "the forces of ethnic biology." Thus, they wanted industrial social workers to be "agents obligated to the community," largely independent of management and the workings of the factory.[194] The employers sought to avert the influence of public biological supervision on their utilization of the female labor force, whether the demand was made in the name of the "State," the "common welfare," or the National Socialist "community." They resisted not only the external source of the demands, but also the social workers' objectives of adapting factory work to the childbearing capacity of the female labor force and the special needs of married women and mothers.

Individual instruction by the Party or DAF was necessary for a minority of employers in order to achieve a thinning out and reorganization of the industrial work force according to racial criteria. To the extent that these criteria supplied a useful tool, the entrepreneurs had long since adopted them. Since workers generally resisted being integrated into the contemporary "industrial community," the industrialists had long been interested in the plant welfare training of a core of workers, family organized and committed to industry, according to such criteria as: "responsible," "healthy," "competent," "permanent," "loyal." The racial conceptions of

the industrialists did not vary significantly from those of the
National Socialists. Nevertheless, the interests of industrial "selection" could often collide with the "breeding" policies of the
"national community" (*Volksgemeinschaft*). After the outbreak of
the war, as might have been suspected, the industrialists, who
already advocated the modern concept of women's dual burden in
both home and factory, would welcome the general conscription of
women into the factories and the integration of women into
industrial production.

During the period of war preparations the industrialists had called
in vain for a universal system of mandatory service by women, and
after the outbreak of the war their representatives in the Reich
Economic Council renewed these demands. But after conscription
was put into effect, the industrialists' experience with conscripted
women workers confirmed their earlier belief in an industrial
practice which depended on maintaining women's double burden by
means both of wages policy and of social and family policy.

Above all, conscripted women—whether unemployed or transferred from other jobs—turned out to be unresponsive to wage
inducements. Those who had chosen to work in offices or department stores in order to increase household income, or who subsisted
on part-time work, were not prepared to wear themselves out
working long days in an armaments factory for a small increase in
income. Moreover, it was less and less worthwhile to work for
money because of the rationing of all necessities, which more or less
precluded a rise in consumption. Instead of using up shoes and
clothing in pointless factory work and handing over ration coupons
for tasteless canteen meals, it made more sense to repair old clothes
and resole shoes at home (the instructions were in the NS-
Frauenwarte) and to stay at home to cultivate vegetables, keep
chickens and rabbits on the balcony, or just generally have time for
"provisioning." Whether women actually believed in the final
victory or not, if they wanted to live through the end of the war they
had to wage a day-to-day struggle for survival. In the factory there
was little for them to gain, but much to lose. The time and strength
which they so urgently needed to organize the working day for
themselves and their dependents was nowhere so rigidly restricted
as in the area of armaments production.

In fact, women preferred *any* office job or unpaid volunteer
position at the NSV or the Red Cross to the paid labor of the factory.
The conscripted women would have given up factory jobs or

exchanged them for non-factory work if exchange had not been forbidden. Most of all, they would have preferred to be released.

The industrialists developed predictable responses to these attitudes. First, as far as personnel requirements and the goodwill of the Labor Office would allow, they avoided hiring conscripted women, falling back instead on foreign labor, male and female. When women employees were finally placed in their industries, they were subjected to the control system in which the industrial social workers played a part. Instead of offering higher wages, companies attempted to motivate women to increase production by using a bonus system: they distributed chocolate and coffee, basing allowances on the difficulty and length of the work assignment, night work, and pregnancy. The extra rations were vital for women, and still more for their children, to whom the rations were often relinquished, because many were not sufficiently nourished by the "normal" rations. Employers also declined, whenever possible, to employ "unsuitable" workers, and they refused to invest more than the absolute minimum in their training.

As for the industrial social workers, the pressures of war, Party, and management demands forced them to abandon, or at least modify, some of their original goals and reasons for being. They had their hands full aiding women whose lives after full-time factory work consisted of endless shopping lines, housework, childcare, and nights in the bomb shelter. In this environment there was scarcely time for education courses and training women in the work ethic. No interest—not the industrialists, the Party, or the social workers themselves—saw its goals for industrial social work completely realized.

Notes

1. Frieda Wunderlich, *Fabrikpflege. Ein Beitrag zur Betriebspolitik* (Berlin, 1926), 12. Dr. Wunderlich (1887–1965), a social scientist, member of the Berlin City Council, 1926–33, for the SPD (Social Democratic Party), professor at the Professional Educational Institute of the Handelshochschule, Berlin, and Editor of *Soziale Praxis*. After her emigration in 1933, she was at the New School for Social Research in New York.

2. Ludwig von Friedeburg, *Betriebsklima. Eine industriesoziologische Untersuchung aus dem Ruhrgebiet unter der wissenschaftlichen Leitung von Ludwig v. Friedeburg*, vol. 3 *Frankfurter Beiträge zur Soziologie*, ed. Theodor W. Adorno and Walter Dirks. (Frankfurt am Main, 1955). For an evaluation of these and following studies see: Burkhardt Lutz and Gert Schmidt, "Industriesoziologie," in *Handbuch der empirischen Sozialforschung*, ed. René König (Stuttgart, 1977) 8:156ff.

3. "Die Werksfürsorgerin bei Bosch," in Robert Bosch Gmbtt (ed.), *Sozialpolitik bei Bosch*, Bosch Publication Series, 4 (Stuttgart, 1951), 89. This self-denying character of industrial welfare work runs through all the articles and statements about their practical experience by industrial social workers from 1900 onward and was turned against them. Edith Zundel, in a recent sociological investigation of social work in industry, discovered that the direct supervisors of the social workers valued the work of these women less than the other personnel did, who placed social counseling in the upper third of a graduated scale of industrial social achievement. Edith Zundel, "Sozialarbeit im Betrieb," *Kölner Zeitschrift für Soziologie und Sozialpsychologie*, 2 (1972): 292, 294, 297ff. See also Margarethe Girmes, *Die Sozialarbeiterin im Industriebetrieb. Versuch einer soziologischen Positionsanalyse* (Weinheim, 1970).

4. On labor and industrial law under National Socialism see: Wolfgang Spohn, "Betriebsgemeinschaft und innerbetriebliche Herrschaft," in Carola Sachse, Tilla Siegel, Hasso Spode, Wolfgang Spohn, *Angst, Belohnung, Zucht und Ordnung. Herrschaftsmechanismen im Nationalsozialismus* (Opladen, 1982), 140–208.

5. Compare the relevant journals: *NS-Frauenwarte* 1 (1932–33), 7 (1943) and *Die Frau am Werk* 1 (1936), 6 (1941) and *Monatshefte für NS-Sozialpolitik*, (1933/34), 10 (1943).

6. See also: Tilla Siegel, "Thesen zur Charakterisierung faschistischer Herrschaft." "Faschismus heute?" *Asthetik und Kommunikation* 32 (June, 1978): 59–70.

7. See the classic studies of Ernst Fraenkel, *Der Doppelstaat* (Frankfurt am Main, 1974) and Franz L. Neumann, *Behemoth. Struktur und Praxis des Nationalsozialismus 1933–1944* (Cologne, 1977) and the current controversy as documented in *Der "Führerstaat." Mythos und Realität. Studien zur Struktur and Politik des Dritten Reiches*, eds. G. Hirschfeld and Lothar Kettenacker (Stuttgart, 1981).

8. A recent monographic discussion of the DAF is not available; therefore see Hans-Gerd Schumann, *Nationalsozialismus und Gewerkschaftsbewegung. Die Vernichtung der deutschen Gewerkschaften und der Aufbau der "Deutschen Arbeitsfront"* (Hannover, 1958) and Timothy W. Mason, *Sozialpolitik im Dritten Reich* (Opladen, 1977).

9. There is a broad spectrum of literature on wage work by women: Dörte Winkler, *Frauenarbeit im "Dritten Reich"* (Hamburg, 1977); Jill Stephenson, *Women in Nazi Society* (London, 1975); Stefan Bajohr, *Die Hälfte der Fabrik. Geschichte der Frauenarbeit in Deutschland 1914–1945* (Marburg, 1979); Renate Bridenthal: "Beyond Kinder, Küche, Kirche: Weimar Women at Work," *Central European History* 6 (1972): 148–66; Gabriele Wellner, "Industriearbeiterinnen in der Weimarer Republik: Arbeitsmarkt, Arbeit und Privatleben 1919–1933," *Geschichte und Gesellschaft* vol. 7, nos. 3/4 (1981): 534–54; see

also in the same volume: Ute Frevert, "Traditionale Weiblichkeit und moderne Interes-senorganisation": 507–33. More concise is the literature on housework and the so-called "private lives" of women; see Gisela Bock, "Frauen und ihre Arbeit im Nationalsozialismus," in *Frauen in der Geschichte*, (Düsseldorf, 1979) vol. 1, eds. Annette Kuhn and Gerhard Schneider; Karin Hausen, "Mütter zwischen Geschäftsinteresse und kultischer Verehrung," in *Sozialgeschichte der Freizeit*, ed. Gerhard Huck (Wuppertal, 1981); Susanna Dammer, "Kinder, Küche Kriegsarbeit. Die nationalsozialistische Schulung der Frauen in der NS-Frauenschaft," in *Mutterkreuz und Arbeitsbuch*, Frauengruppe Faschismusforschung (Frankfurt, 1982). See also in the same volume: Annemarie Tröger, "Die Frau im wesensgemässen Einsatz."

10. Gertrud Scholtz-Klink. (b. 1902) worked in the Red Cross. In 1928 she became a member of the NSDAP and began her party career as a women's labor service leader in Württemberg. In 1934 she became Reich Women's Leader in a merger of the leadership of the National Socialist Women's Organization, German Women's Work, the Women's Bureau of the DAF, and the Women's Labor Service, (later the Reich service for young women). In 1945, she was arrested for war crimes and classified as a "major offender." She was acquitted, and released in 1949.

11. Current work in oral history is helping to fill this gap. I am especially grateful for the research of Irmgard Weyrather and Christl Wickert. The debate over industrial social work in the 'twenties was documented in contemporary journals. See especially: *Der Arbeitgeber. Zeitschrift der Vereinigung der Deutschen Arbeitgeberverbände*, (1904–1934); *Die Arbeit. Zeitschrift für Gewerkschaftspolitik und Wirtschaftskunde*, edited by Theodor Leipart, 1924–1933; *Die Frau. Monatsschrift für das gesamte Frauenleben unserer Zeit*. Founded by Helene Lange and edited by Gertrud Baumer and Frances Magnus von Hausen, 1893–94 to 1943–44; *Soziale Praxis und Archiv für Volkswohlfahrt*, earlier edited by Ernst Francke in 1922, edited by Ludwig Heyde, 1891–92 to 1944 and subsequently appearing as *Die deutsche Sozialpolitik. Gemeinschaftsarbeit der Zeitschrift "Soziale Praxis" und "Monatshefte für NS Sozialpolitik"* zugleich Kriegsausgabe der Zeitschrift Soziale Zukunft, 1944–45 (Organ of the Society for Social Reform); *Nachrichtendienst des Vereins für öffentliche und private Fürsorge* (1920–1941); *Die Arbeiterwohlfahrt*. Committee for Workers' Welfare (1926–1933).

A few monographs, for the most part written by plant welfare workers, discussed the practice of industrial social work; see: Margarete Grundies, "Bericht aus der Werksfürsorge-Arbeit" *Kindergarten* 72 (1931): 199–204; Gertrud Henseleit, "Die Fabrikpflege und ihre Interes-senten," *Soziale Praxis und Archiv für Volkswohlfahrt* vol. 35 no. 48 (1926): col. 1227–1235;

Ludwig Schmidt-Kehl, *Die deutsche Fabrikpflegerin* (Berlin, 1926); Wunderlich, *Fabrikpflege*. Rudolf Schwenger also describes factory welfare in detail: *Die betriebliche Sozialpolitik im Ruhrkohlenbergbau*, and *Die betriebliche Sozialpolitik in der westdeutschen Grosseisenindustrie*, parts 1 and 2 of *Die betriebliche Sozialpolitik einzelner Industriezweige*, Goetz Briefs (Munich, 1932–34) (*Schriften des Vereins fur Sozialpolitik*, 186). The material pertinent to this article is located in large part in the German Central Institute for Social Problems (Deutsches Zentralinstitut für Soziale Fragen), Berlin-Dahlem. It is catalogued there under "Werksfürsorge."

Industrial positions that diverged from DAF policy can be gleaned from scattered references and industrial measures. See records of the Werner-von-Siemens-Institut, Munich [cited as Siemens Archivakte and Aktensignatur (SAA)]. Mrs. Lenore Riedrich, former Leader of the Social Counseling Division at the Siemens plant in Munich, made several other documents available to me—notably "Industrial Welfare" excerpts from the yearly reports of the Social/Political Division of the Siemens plant, collected by Brigitta Einehr in 1949 (cited as Siemens-Jahresbericht . . . " and year; Records of the Bundesarchiv (BA) Koblenz R 12I

(Reichsgruppe Industrie), R 13 Wirtschaftsgruppen Reichsgruppe Industrie, NS 5I (Deutsche Arbeitsfront).

12. There is no comprehensive portrayal of the history of industrial social policy in Germany. Older works, better used as sources for a general understanding of industrial sociology than as empirical studies, are: L.H.A. Geck, *Die sozialen Arbeitsverhältnisse im Wandel der Zeit*, (Berlin, 1931; revised ed. Darmstadt, 1977); Ernst Michel, *Sozialgeschichte der industriellen Arbeitswelt* (Frankfurt am Main, 1948). Only cash concerns in the nineteenth century have been historically researched: Ludwig Puppke, "Sozialpolitik und soziale Anschauungen frühindustrieller Unternehmer in Rheinland-Westfalen" (Dissertation; Cologne, 1966); Günter Schulz, "Fabriksparkassen für Arbeiter. Konzeption und Inanspruchnahme einer betrieblichen Institution," *Zeitschrift für Unternehmensgeschichte* vol. 25, no. 3 (1980): 145–78. In addition see Gerhard Adelmann (ed.), *Quellensammlung zur Geschichte der sozialen Betriebsverfassung. Ruhrindustrie unter besonderer Berücksichtigung des Industrie-und Handelskammerbezirks Essen. Publikation der Gesellschaft für Rheinische Geschichtskunde LIV* (1960–1968).

13. For a discussion of educational plans see: Alice Salomon, *Leitfaden de Wohlfahrtspflege*, (Berlin, 1923) and *Richtlinien für die Lehrpläne der Wohlfahrtsschulen*, Prussian Ministry of Public Welfare (Berlin, 1930). This contains introductions by Alice Salomon, Maria Offenberg, and Elisabeth Nitzsche. The Soziale Museum in Frankfurt am Main organized conferences on plant policy, see *Soziale Praxis* 33 (924): col. 644ff; 35 (1926): col. 627ff; 39 (1930): col. 1167ff. In 1925, an International Congress for Industrial Welfare took place in Vlissingen. Compare Hildegard Böhme, "Neue Wege der Betriebswohlfahrtspflege," *Die Frau*, vol. 33 no. 1 (1925): 39–43; Frieda Wunderlich reported about this in *Soziale Praxis* vol. 36, no. 28 (1925): col. 617–919. For discussion of the international aspects see Alice Salomon, "Industrielle Wohlfahrt als neue Philosophie," *Soziale Praxis* vol. 31, no. 43 (1932): col. 1171–1174; Margarete Kaiser-Harnisch, "Fabrikpflege auf wirtschaftspsychologischer Grundlage," *Die Arbeit* vol. 2, no. 12 (1925): 774–76; and, "Der Stand der Fabrikpflegebewegung," *Die Arbeit* vol. 3, no. 4 (1926): 266ff; also see unsigned article in *Soziale Praxis* 33 (1924): col. 592; 34 (1925): col. 42–44.

14. For the current data see Lenor Riedrich, *Von der Werksfürsorge zur Sozialberatung* (Essen, 1976), 8; and her "Betriebliche Sozialarbeit in der Spannung zwischen wirtschaftlichen Abläufen und menschlichen Problemen," *Blätter der Wohlfahrtspflege* 7 (1977): 148–51.

15. Ludwig Puppke, "Sozialpolitik und soziale Anschauungen frühindustrieller Unternehmer in Rheinland-Westfalen" (Dissertation: Cologne, 1966), 209–13.

16. See Dr. J. Altenrath, "Vorbericht," in *Aufgabe und Organisation der Fabrikwohlfahrtspflege in der Gegenwart, Vorbericht und Verhandlungen der 4. Konferenz der Zentralstelle für Volkswohlfahrt am 6. Juni in Braunschweig* (Berlin, 1910), 1–176, esp. 117–131; Dr. Czimatis, "Empfiehlt es sich, auf die Einstellung von sog. Fabrikpflegerinnen hinzuwirken?" *Concordia* vol. 16, no. 1: 11–15; L. Katscher, *Sozialsekretäre und Fabrikpfleger* (Leipzig, 1907); Elisabeth Altmann-Gottheiner, "Die Fabrikpflegerin," *Blätter für Soziale Arbeit* vol. 9 no. 4, (1917): 21–24; an historical overview is given by Margarete Cordemann, *Werksfürsorge*, Archiv für Wohlfahrtspflege, (today Deutsches Zentralinstitut für soziale Fragen), (Berlin, 1955). For the story of the founding of the Women's Social Work School, see Alice Salomon, *Leitfaden der Wohlfahrtspflege* (Berlin, 1923), 164; see also Maria Pauls, *Die deutschen Frauenorganisationen. Eine Übersicht über den Bestand, die Ursprünge und die kulturellen Aufgaben* (Dissertation: Aachen, 1966, p. 133).

17. Marie-Elisabeth Lüders. *Das unbekannte Heer* (Berlin, 1936). 199ff.

18. Lüders, *Heer*, 120, 135, 137. Dr. Marie-Elisabeth Lüders (1878–1966) was a home-care worker in Berlin-Charlottenburg in 1912–15; after 1916 she was the Director of the FAZ. She was a member of the National Assembly in 1919 and DDP Member of the Reichstag, 1920–33. She was imprisoned for six months in 1937 and was forbidden to work or publish. From 1948 to 1950 she was a city representative in Berlin, from 1949 to 1961 FDP Bundestag member.

On factory social service in the First World War see also Charlotte Lorenz, "Die gewerbliche Frauenarbeit während des Krieges," in Paul Umbreit, *Der Krieg und die Arbeitsverhältnisse*. *Wirtschafts-und Sozialgeschichte des Weltkriegs*, Carnegie Foundation for International Peace, Deutsche Serie (Stuttgart, New Haven, 1928), 307–391, especially 366ff. In the preparatory phases of the Second World War there was an intensified interest in the war experience of factory welfare programs which manifested itself in a number of publications on this topic: Irmgard Fischer, "Aus meinem Kriegstagebuch als Fabrikpflegerin in den Dillinger Hüttenwerken," in *Nationalsozialistische Mädchenerziehung*, 1935, no. 11, p. 335–338; Lüders, *Heer*, and "Fabrikpflege," in *Die Frau* 5 (1936): 262–76; Theodor Sonnemann; *Die Frau in der Landesverteidigung und ihr Einsatz in der Industrie* (Oldenburg, 1939), 145. For a newer presentation see Ursula v. Gersdorff, *Frauen im Kriegsdienst* (Stuttgart, 1969), 15ff; also "Frauenarbeit und Frauenemanzipation im Ersten Weltkrieg," *Francia* 2 (1975): 502–23.

19. See Lüders, *Heer*, 187; Wunderlich, *Fabrikpflege*, 5; Lorenz, *Frauenarbeit*, 366ff.

20. Henseleit, *Fabrikpflege*, col. 1231: "The war economy hardly needed to worry about profitability. That humanity was very much elevated by the war appears to me to be, at the least, hypothetical."

21. In *Blätter für Soziale Arbeit* vol. 9, no. 6 (1917): 36ff, under the heading "Women's Social Work Schools" the founding of two new schools is reported and also recent "warnings against further foundings of Social Work Schools." See Margarete Cordemann, *Wie es wirklich gewesen ist. Lebenserinnerungen einer Sozialarbeiterin auf dem Hintergrund der Beschreibung der deutschen Gesellschaft in der Zeit von 1890–1960* (Gladbeck, 1963).

22. "Ausbildung von Fabrikpflegerinnen," *Blätter für Soziale Arbeit* vol. 9, no. 6 (1917): 37ff; "Schreiben des Verbandes katholischer Vereine erwerbstätiger Frauen und Mädchen Deutschlands," Berlin, February 1917, in von Gersdorff, *Kriegsdienst* (1969), 146ff; Lüders, *Fabrikpflege*, 265–66. Wunderlich, *Fabrikpflege*, 16, on the other hand, believed that all of the trained social workers were already employed in War Office positions, so that women who "did not always [fit] the ideal aptitudes" had to be hired: thus the mass lay-offs of factory social service workers after the war.

23. Calculated from Lorenz' data, *Frauenarbeit*, 348 and Wunderlich, *Fabrikpflege*, 6; Lüders (*Heer*, 85, 188) reports the high point as 900 factory social service workers in October 1918; some factory social service workers were responsible for several factories. In all about 2.1 million women were employed in industry.

24. See Lüders *Heer*, 190ff, 197–207; Fischer, *Kriegstagebuch*; Wunderlich, *Fabrikpflege*, 13ff; Anneliese Seidel, *Frauenarbeit im Ersten Weltkrieg als Problem der staatlichen Sozialpolitik. Dargestellt am Beispiel Bayerns*. (Frankfurt am Main, 1979), 160–71.

25. Wunderlich, *Fabrikpflege*, 14; von Gerdsoff, *Kriegsdienst*, 34f; Schmidt-Kehl, *Fabrikpflegerin*, 36.

26. Annemarie Tröger, "Die Dolchstosslegende. der Linken: 'Frauen haber Hitler an die Macht gebracht,'" *Frauen und Wissenschaft, Beiträge zur Berliner Sommeruniversität für Frauen Juli 1976* (Berlin, 1977).

27. This was a crucial problem in the nineteenth century, especially in the Ruhr area, where the workforce consisted mainly of recent immigrants from other regions of Germany.

28. Wunderlich, *Fabrikpflege*, 8–10; Schmidt-Kehl, *Fabrikpflegerin*, 23–25. *Die Blätter der Wohlfahrtspflege* vol. 124, no. 7 (1977) discussed this problem of industrial social workers, as immediate now as it was then, under the title "Zwischen allen Stühlen." (Falling Between the Stools.)

29. The numbers given for factory social service workers are extremely variable and cannot be completely reconstructed: Schmidt-Kehl, *Fabrikpflegerin*, 7, reports for 1925 110 factory social service workers in 116 factories; apparently, there were another 41 plant welfare workers in the Ruhr district in 1926 (see Schwenger, *Ruhrkohlenbergbau*, 167); Henseleit, *Fabrikpflege*, 1231 reports 80–90 factory social service workers for the year

1926. The difference can be partly explained by the fact that some authors include factory nurses.

30. Schwenger, *Ruhrkohlenbergbau*, 162f. See Lüders *Heer*, 182, 172, 125, 115 ("Vergiftung völkischen Lebenskraft") and 63ff; see also Sonnemann, *Landesverteidigung*, 131; Cordemann (*Lebenserinnerungen*, 193) also complained about the serious "spiritual devastation" that the war had caused among women, without, however, seeing the national danger.

31. Schwenger, *Ruhrkohlenbergbau*, 162f.

32. Grundies, *Werksfürsorge*, 203f.

33. Peter C. Bäumer, "Das Deutsche Institut für technische Arbeitsschulung (1930)," in *Probleme der sozialen Werkspolitik. Schriften des Vereins für Sozialpolitik*, 181, part 1 (Munich, 1930–35). 90.

34. We need a history of the Kaleidoscopic expression "from help to self-help" as it was variously used by the Prussian prison reformers, the workers' movement, the women's movement, the social policy makers of the Weimar Republic, and finally the National Socialists, and what each meant by it.

35. See Grundies, *Werksfürsorge*, 201. On the factory domestic education courses in the German monarchy, see Gerda Tornierporth, *Studien zur Frauenbildung* (Weinheim, 1979), 123–40.

36. Schwenger, *Ruhrkohlenbergbau*, 180; Bäumer, *DINTA*, 90; Grundies, *Werksfürsorge*, 201.

37. Schmidt-Kehl, *Fabrikpflegerin*, 16–18; Wunderlich, *Fabrikpflege*, 26.

38. Schwenger, *Ruhrkohlenbegbau*, 157ff, 174–82, and his *Grosseisenindustrie*, 128–33, lists the "Zeche ver. Stein-Hardenberg der Bergbau Gruppe Dortmund der Vereinigten Stahlwerke AG," the Victoria-Lünen mines of the Harpener Berbau-AG, the Gutehoffnungsnütte; in all, domestic economy courses were held at over 30 mining centers in the Ruhr district; for the iron and steel industry the Friedrich-Krupp-AG and the August-Thyssen-Hütte are given.

39. Grundies, *Werksfürsorge*, 201.

40. Ibid., 199ff.

41. Schwenger, *Ruhrkohlenbergbau*, 163.

42. R. Michels: *Psychologie der antikapitalistichen Massenbewegungen (Grundriss der Sozialökonomik* vol 9, part 1), 333ff, cited in Bäumer, *DINTA*, 89. The leader of DINTA, Karl Arnhold, specifically refers to Michels, see Grundies, *Werksfürsorge*, 203, and Gerhard P. Bunk, *Erziehung und Industriearbeit* (Weinheim, 1972), 223, 259. K. Arnhold (1884–1970), Head Engineer, was a technical teacher in Wuppertal before the First World War. After 1921 he developed the educational system of the Schalker Verein of the Gelsenkirchener Bergwerks-AG. Leader of DINTA, supported by the Verein deutscher Eisenhüttenleute, founded in 1925. DINTA was absorbed by the DAF in 1934–35 as "Amt für Berufserziehung und soziale Betriebsführung," still under the leadership of Arnhold. After the end of the war, he ran the Gesellschaft für Arbeitspädagogik mbH in Witten/Ruhr, which advised employers. In 1960 he was awarded the Bundesverdienstkreuz First Class. See Bunk, *Erziehung*, 259ff.

43. Respectively Grundies, *Werksfürsorge*, 202, 203; Schwenger, *Ruhrkohlenbergbau*, 174, 179; Bäumer, *DINTA*, 90. Margarete Grundies was the director of factory welfare in the Gelsenkirchener Bergwerks-AG in Dortmund and draws in her work on the ideas of DINTA.

44. Grundies, *Werksfürsorge*, 201; see also Schwenger, *Ruhrkohlenbergbau*, 175; "care of the home" was supposed to lead to "a suitable standard of domestic taste."

45. Schwenger, *Grosseisenindustrie*, 133–36.

46. Schwenger, *Ruhrkohlenbergbau*, 174, 179.

47. Schmidt-Kehl, *Fabrikpflege*, 16.

48. Grundies, *Werksfürsorge*. 203; see also Bunk, *Erziehung*, 223; Peter Hinrichs and Lothar Peter, *Industrielle Friede? Arbeitswissenschaft, Rationalisierung und Arbeiterbewegung in der Weimarer Republik* (Köln, 1976), 73; Bäumer, *DINTA*, 90; Schwenger,

Ruhrkohlenbergbau, 174. That this line of reasoning was spread beyond DINTA, if less drastically formulated, is shown by Ludwig Preller, "Fabrikpflege und Wohlfahrtspflege," *Arbeiterwohlfahrt* vol. 2, no. 7 (1927), 196. Dr. Ludwig Preller (1897–1973) was an editor of *Soziale Praxis* and a member of the SPD and ADGB (the German Trade Union Federation). From 1926–33 he was a senior civil servant in the Reich Ministry of Labor and in the Saxon Ministry of Welfare and Labor; he was dismissed in 1933, and then became director of the department "Social Legislation and Social Affairs" in the (state-run) Textile Industry Economic Group in Berlin (BA Koblenz, R 13 XIV/54: Protokoll über eine Besprechung am 1. und 2.2 1944): from 1948 to 1950, he was Minister for Labor, Business, and Transportation in Schleswig-Holstein; later he was a member of the Bundestag. See also Wunderlich, *Fabrikpflege*, 30.

49. Along with Ilse Ganzert, Lotte Jahn (later Salm) was an initiator of "industrial social work." Jahn came from a pastor's family. She may have "imagined that the Commission for Industrial Social Work could take on the role of an evangelical deaconess and thus go beyond the economic security of industrial social workers by providing them with spiritual and moral support." At least it was so speculated in the Reichsgruppe Industrie in 1935; see *BA Koblenz*, R 12/252: Studders (member of Reichsgruppe Industrie) to Dr. Trendelenburg (1935–36, Director of the Reichsgruppe Industrie), on August 31, 1935. Lotte Jahn was a social industrial worker at Oetker (Bielefeld) until 1938 and was responsible there for women interns training to become industrial social workers. (*BA Koblenz* NS 5 I/219: Aktenvermerk vom June 20, 1939). Ilse Ganzert was, like Lotte Jahn, a member of the ADGB. Whether her activity in it went beyond simple membership could not be established; her theme was "to win the trust of the female staff." At this time she spoke "very strongly against the then still purely industry-led DINTA." In 1934 she became a specialist for industrial social work in the Women's Bureau of the DAF and worked in this function closely with the DINTA which had then been taken over by the DAF. Further personal data for either woman were not found.

50. Wunderlich, *Fabrikpflege*, 25.

51. Henseleit, *Fabrikpflege*, col. 1232.

52. Ibid., col. 1229.

53. Ibid., 1230; "Kriegsaufgaben in der Fürsorge für die werktätigen Menschen" *Nachrichtendienst des Deutschen Vereins für öffentliche und private Fürsorge* vol. 20, no. 10, (1939): 303.

54. Ilse Ganzert, "Soziale Betriebsarbeit," *Die Frau* 6 (1929): 343.

55. Ganzert, "Soziale Betriebsarbeit," 345.

56. Lotte Salm, "Soziale Betriebsarbeit," *Arbeiterwohlfahrt* vol. 5 no. 15 (1930): 454.

57. Wunderlich, *Fabrikpflege*, 32.

58. Ilse Ganzert, "Soziale Betriebsarbeit," *Neue Blätter für den Sozialismus* vol. 1 no. 5 (1930): 217; a year before the author had still recognized that "wearing, mechanized piece work left open the possibility of personal development within industrial work only for a very few, isolated cases." Ganzert, "Soziale Betriebsarbeit" (1929), 342.

59. Ibid., 346, 342, 344, 348; see also her "Soziale Betriebsarbeit" (1930), 215, 217; Salm, "Soziale Betriebsarbeit," 455.

60. Ganzert, "Soziale Betriebsarbeit" (1930), 216–18.

61. Hendrik de Man, *Der Kampf um die Arbeitsfreude. Eine Untersuchung auf Grund der Aussagen von 78 Industriearbeitern und Angestellten* (Jena, 1927). Hendrik de Man (1885–1953) was a Lecturer at the (Trade Union) Akademie der Arbeit in Frankfurt in the 1920s; from 1933–41, he was a Professor in Brussels. In 1939 he became the President of the Belgian Workers' Party. In 1941 he left Belgium after the failure of an attempted collaboration with the German occupation. In 1946 he was sentenced in absentia (Swiss exile) to twenty years in prison.

62. Grundies, *Werksfürsorge*, 202 ff.

63. Ganzert, "Soziale Betriebsarbeit" (1930); Wunderlich, *Fabrikpflege*, 26; Grundies, *Werksfürsorge*, 200.

64. Ganzert, "Soziale Betriebsarbeit" (1929), 345, 347; Salm, "Soziale Betriebsarbeit," 456.

65. *BA Koblenz* R 121/252, Consultation Studders/Ganzert on Sept 1, 1931 and Studders to Trendelenburg on August 31, 1935; *BA Koblenz*, R 12 I/253, minutes of a consultation with representatives of coal mining concerning social work in the firm, October 28, 1937 by the representatives of the Reichsgruppe Industrie.

66. Gertrud Hanna, "Noch einmal: Soziale Betriebsarbeit. Eine Erwiderung," *Arbeiterwohlfahrt* vol. 5, no. 15 (1930): 457–460; and her "Werksfürsorge und Wohlfahrtspflege," *Arbeiterwohlfahrt* vol. 5 no. 7 (1930): 193–202. Gertrud Hanna (1876–1944), a print shop assistant, became the secretary of the women workers' committee and in 1916 took over the editorship of the *Gewerkschaftliche Frauenzeitung*. She was a SPD representative to the Prussian Landtag until 1933. In 1944 she committed suicide. Schmidt-Kehl, *(Fabrikpflegerin*, 23) reported "distrust" among the "more or less radical part of the workers": see also Wunderlich, *Fabrikpflege*, 9.

67. Heimann, "Soziale Betriebsarbeit," *Neue Blätter für den Sozialismus* vol. 1, no. 5 (1930): 226. "And when one considers that factory welfare workers are almost only active in predominantly female industries . . . and that it is exactly among women that lack of interest in the factory as a whole is most pronounced, one can imagine that a factory council member who takes his duty seriously must welcome a fellow struggler against the enemy: lack of interest and indifference." Eduard Heimann (1889–1967) was a professor of economics and the sociology of religion. He was coeditor of the *Neue Blätter für den Sozialismus*, a journal of protestant socialism. He emigrated to New York in 1933 and was at the New School for Social Research. On trade union conflicts with DINTA, see Fritz Fricke, *Sie suchen die Seele!* (Berlin, 1927); also *Dintageist—Wirtschaftsbürger. Eine Streitschrift*, (Köln, 1950); see also Wunderlich, *Fabrikpflege*, 29.

68. Salm, "Soziale Betriebsarbeit," 457.

69. SAA/DAF-SB, undated (circa summer 1942) internal document probably written by Burhenne (Siemens—Social Policy Department).

70. Otto Marrenbach ed., *Fundamente des Sieges. Die Gesamtarbeit der Deutschen Arbeiterfront von 1933 bis 1940*, (Berlin, 1940), 239.

71. Ganzert, "Soziale Betriebsarbeit" (1929); similarly, Ingeborg Claussen, "Die Aufgaben der Sozialen Betriebsarbeiterin," *Die Ärztin* 6 (1941): 249.

72. Compare with the autobiographical reports of two women who were active in the BDM and the Reichsarbeitsdienst: Renate Finckh, *Mit uns zieht die neue Zeit*, (Baden-Baden, 1979); Melitta Maschmann, *Fazit. Mein Weg in die Hitler-Jugend*. (Munich, 1979; first ed. Stuttgart, 1963).

73. *BA Koblenz*, R 12 I/252, "Betr. Soziale Betriebsarbeit" Brochure of the DAF Women's Bureau of October 8, 1935. The factory leader and representative were to confirm that they had "placed in leadership" the appropriate woman worker. Ilse Reiche, "Die Soziale Betriebsarbeiterin," *Die Frau* vol. 44, no. 9 (1937): 489. Rudolf Bethmann, "Betriebswohlfahrtspflege—Soziale Betriebsarbeit," *Zentralblatt für Gewerbehygiene und Unfallverhütung* vol. 22, no. 10 (1935) (new series, vol. 12): 177. The history of the Women's Schools is not yet written. Some are mentioned in Cordemann, *Lebenserinnerungen* and Pauls, *Frauenorganisationen*. In Berlin, the Deutsche Akademie für soziale und pädagogische Frauenarbeit, under the direction of Alice Salomon, was dissolved by the National Socialists, as well as the Verein Jugendheim in Charlottenburg directed by Anna von Gierke: see also the brochure: *Anna von Gierke. Zum 100 Geburtstag. 14 März 1974*, produced by the Berliner Frauenbund 1945 e.V.

74. Anna Maria Hanne (later Hanne-Braun) was an agent of the Women's Bureau in the DAF and later the deputy leader to the Reich Women's Leader Scholtz-Klink, in charge of industrial social work. Further personal data could not be found.

75. Marrenbach, *Fundamente, 239; BA Koblenz*, R 12 I/252; Studders to Trendelenburg on August 21, 1935; Circular letter from Arnhold (Leader of the DINTA in the DAF) on

October 8, 1934; Scholtz-Klink to Hecker (1934–35 president of Reichswirtschaftskammer) on July 22, 1935.

76. *BA Koblenz*, R 12 I/252: "Soziale Betriebsarbeit," October 28, 1935 (brochure). The amount of the social industrial workers' salaries is not known to me. The salaries of the plant welfare workers who were independent of the DAF and paid directly by the employer were between 200 and 230 Reichsmark (starting salary) and 300 and 400 RM, and in some cases significantly more; BA Koblenz, R 12 I/252, Studders to Dierig (Textile manufacturer from Langenbielau and temporary Reichswirtschaftsrat in 1934–35) November 27, 1935.

77. Ibid., among others. The following firms employed DAF industrial social workers: New York-Hamburger Gummiwaren & Co.; Greiff-Werke, AG Greifenberg/Schlesien; Promota-Chemische Fabrik, Hamburg; Oetker, Bielefeld; see letter from Studders to Vielmetter (General Director of Knorr-Bremse, Berlin) October 14, 1935. For statistics see Bethmann, "Betriebswohlfahrtspflege," 176; all statistics on industrial social work are to be used with caution, as official statistics were not maintained and every author defined and included or excluded factory nurses, kindergarten teachers, and plant welfare workers according to his or her own criteria.

78. Ibid., Pfotenhauer (or Merck, Darmstadt) to the Reichswirtschaftskammer October 3, 1935; Firma Henkel (Düsseldorf) to the Reichsgruppe Industrie, October 29, 1935. On the "Organisation der gewerblichen Wirtschaft" see Karl Guth, *Die Reichsgruppe Industrie* (Berlin, 1941); Ingeborg Esenwein-Rothe, *Die Wirtschaftsverbände von 1933 bis 1945* (Berlin, 1965).

79. *BA Koblenz*, R 12 I/252: Dierig to Reichsgruppe Industrie, October 15, 1935.

80. Ibid.: Reichsgruppe Industrie to Reichswirtschaftskammer, October 30, 1935.

81. Ibid.: *Sozialarbeit im Betrieb* (brochure), December 11, 1935. Text of the agreement between the Reichswirtschaftskammer, Reichsgruppe Industrie and the DAF on the basis of the discussion of October 28, 1935. See also Marrenbach, *Fundamente*, 240: In addition came internships in the Labor Service, hospital, with the NSV, and with an already active social industrial worker.

82. *BA Koblenz* R 12 I/253: Letter of the Reichsgruppe Industrie of January 17, 1936; Friedrich-Krupp-Germania-Werft to the Reichsgruppe Industrie, April 12, 1936; Letter of the DAF-Gauwaltung Silesia, of June 29, 1936.

83. *BA Koblenz*, R 12 I/253 and 254 contain assorted newspaper clippings referring to this; see also Claussen, "Aufgaben," 250.

84. *BA Koblenz*, R 12 I/253: Gruschwitz-Textilwerke to the Reichsgruppe Industrie, January 6, 1936; Hanne (DAF-Women's Bureau) to the Reichsgruppe Industrie November 10, 1936; Circular letter of the Reichsgruppe Industrie, December 11, 1936. Notes on a discussion between representatives of mining and the Reichsgruppe Industrie, October 28, 1937.

85. Ibid.: DAF-Social Bureau to the Reichsanstalt für Arbeitsvermittlung und Arbeitslosenversicherung, December 18, 1936; Reichsgruppe Industrie to Reichsanstalt, March 24, 1937; Discussion with mining representatives, October 28, 1937.

86. *BA Koblenz*, R 12 I/254: Hanne-Braun (DAF-Women's Bureau) to Lohmann (Secretary of the Reichsgruppe Industrie), June 21, 1939; Hanne-Braun to Lohmann, July 3, 1939; File notation by Lohmann about a discussion with DAF representatives, May 12, 1944; Minutes of the work group "Soziale Betriebsarbeiterin" of the Reichsgruppe Industrie from May 16, 1944; DAF Directive No. . . . /140 Draft (Women's Bureau)/Alternated Draft (Reichsgruppe Industrie) April 14, 1944; Notation on a meeting of the work group "Soziale Betriebsarbeiterin," May 11, 1944.

87. Ibid: Nussbruch (DAF secretariat) to Marten (Special Representative of the Women's Bureau of the DAF staff, Rhein/Ruhr) June 23, 1944; Circular letter from Ganzert (DAF Women's Bureau) July 17, 1944.

88. *Berliner Börsenzeitung* July 30, 1940, SAA/DAF-SB; *BA Koblenz*, R 12 I/263: Hilde Eiserhardt (Association for Public and Private Welfare) to Dr. Reuss (Reichsgruppe

Industrie) July 10, 1939; the same, "Kriegsaufgaben in der Fürsorge für die werktätigen Volksgenossen, III. Fürsorgearbeit in Betrieben mit männlicher und weiblicher Gefolgschaft (Fortsetzung des Artikels "Kriegsaufgaben . . . "") In the Merck company, Darmstadt, factory Women's groups were seen as the "long arm of the welfare worker," especially in "educational and technical welfare." Seven thousand DAF Women's groups had been reorganized by 1943. Gertrud Scholtz-Klink, "Sozialpolitische Aufbauarbeit für die schaffende Frau," *Monatshefte für NS-sozialpolitik* 3–4 (1943): 26; Marrenbach says 3200 (1940); Sonnemann, 500 plant women's groups.

89. *Nachrichtendienst der Reichsfrauenföhrung* vol. 5, no. 1 (January 1936): 43.

90. Sonnemann, *Landesverteidigung*, 148 ff; see also Gertrud Scholtz-Klink, *Die Frau im Dritten Reich. Eine Dokumentation* (Tübingen, 1978), 333; Claussen, "Aufgaben," 251.

91. *BA Koblenz*, R 12 I/253: "Soziale Betriebsarbeit—eine Aufgabe des Frauenamts der deutschen Arbeitsfront" (brochure, circa July/August 1936): relatively young DAF representatives were preferred, women who had been in factory work for at least five years.

92. SAA/DAF-SB: Discussion by mining representatives in the Reichsgruppe Industrie of October 28, 1937. File dated October 27, 1939; *BA Koblenz*, R 12 I/254: Hanne-Braun to Lohmann on June 21, 1939. *Berliner Lokalanzieger*, January 7, 1942. See also Scholtz-Klink, *Frau*, 331.

Year	Number of Industrial Social Workers	Source
1935	410	Bethmann, "Betriebswohlfahrtspflege," 176.
1938	1,000	*Kölnische Volkszeitung*, January 1, 1938, no. 2, *BA Koblenz*, R 12/I/254.
1939	900	*Der Angriff*, April 3, 1941, in SAA/DAF-SB.
1940	1,200	Marrenbach, *Fundamente*, 239.
1941	1,800	*Der Angriff*, January 7, 1942, SAA/DAF-SB.
1942	2,000	*Berliner-Lokalanzeiger*, January 7, 1942, SAA/DAF-SB.
1943	3,000	Scholtz-Klink, *Aufbauarbeit*, 26.*

* These figures probably include plant welfare officers and factory social service workers not recognized as industrial social workers. There are no figures for how many firms employed social workers.

93. *BA Koblenz*, R 12 I/254: Hanne-Braun to Lohmann, June 5, 1939 and June 21, 1939; Dr. Weiss (Social Director at IG-Farben, Ludwigshafen) to Lohmann, June 10, 1939.

94. The DAF Women's Bureau itself had supported this argument as part of the competing Nazi organizations by deferring to the NS People's Welfare and NS Women's Corps from the beginning.

95. *BA Koblenz* R 12 I/254: Agreement between Buskühl (Harpener Mines AG) and Scholtz-Klink, March 28, 1938. *BA Koblenz* R 12 I/253: In discussions between representatives of the mining industry and the Reichsgruppe Industrie on October 28, 1937, the General Director of the Essen Hard Coal mines, Tengelmann, stated: "The mining industry will not allow interference in its affairs. The factory leaders will see to it, even if other branches of industry don't have the courage to defend themselves against the continual attempts to exert external control over the firms."

96. Date	No. of Factory Social Workers	Data For
1924–34	10/11	Metropolitan Berlin
1935–36	14	"
1936–37	16	"
1938–39	24	Germany and Austria
1939–40	25	"
1940–41	30	"
1943	37	"
1945	32	Berlin

Source: Siemens Jahresberichte, 1949.

97. SAA/DAF-SB: Report by two Siemens industrial social workers on a DAF training course, November 2, 1941.

98. SAA/DAF-SB: Entry and file notes on a discussion between Witzleben (Social policy department at Siemens) and Scholtz-Klink, February 26, 1942.

99. The discussion of this is documented in an extended exchange of letters between the Social Policy Department and the DAF Women's Bureau as well as in various internal documents from the years 1939–43, in SAA/DAF-SB.

100. Winkler, *Frauenarbeit*, 78; on industrial social work in general, see 78–81, 159. Winkler also announced here a forthcoming article on the conflict over industrial social work between the employers and the DAF.

101. *BA Koblenz*, R 12 I/253.

102. *BA Koblenz*, R 12 I/267: Seeliger (Director of the Social-Economic Commission of the Reichsgruppe Industrie) to Bieske (apparently an employer in Königsberg). Rough draft of a letter without date (apparently end of 1936). I wish to thank Tilla Siegel for the reference to this document.

103. *BA Koblenz*, R 12 I/253.

104. Ibid., Speech of Scholtz-Klink, May 15, 1936. On occupational organizations see: *Nachrichtendienst der Reichsfrauenführung* vol. 5, no. 2 (1936): 93. I suspect that this separation was later dropped; in later press announcements the definitional difference between plant welfare officers and industrial social workers was no longer made.

105. The Reich convention of factory and plant welfare officers and social service workers in mining was held in May, that of the social industrial workers in October, 1936, see *Nachrichtendienst der Reichsfrauenführung*, vol. 5, no. 5 (1936): 202; no. 11: 416. *BA Koblenz*, R 12 I/253 and 254 contain extensive correspondence about joint training and propaganda trips of Lohmann (Reichsgruppe Industrie) and Hanne (DAF Women's Bureau).

106. *Nachrichtendienst der Reichsfrauenführung*, vol. 5, no. 11 (1936): 416.

107. SAA/DAF-SB: Report from Siemens factory welfare officers on two DAF training courses with a copy of the course program, November 2, 1940; a similar program is contained in *BA Koblenz*, R 12 I/254, Course from January 3–14, 1939. In the same meeting at which Scholtz-Klink gave the speech quoted above, Dr. Bartels (Deputy Reich Medical Leader) also spoke to representatives of industry about the necessity of raising the birthrate: *BA Koblenz*, R 12I/253, May 15, 1936.

108. For educational lectures on "Women's Health" see SAA/DAF-BA: Report on a training course held on February 11, 1940: "Kriegsaufgaben . . . ," 302 ff; Freya Hoesch, "Aufgaben einer Werkpflegeabteilung in der Industrie," *Soziale Praxis* 39 (1935): 1139, 1141; Reiche, "Soziale Betriebsarbeiterin," 490; Oskar Traun, "Die Soziale Betriebsarbeit," *Bericht Weltkongress für Freizeit und Erholung* (Hamburg, July 23–30, 1936), edited by Internationale Zentral-Büro "Freude und Arbeit," Berlin-Hamburg, 1937 212. On consumption management as a task of industrial social workers see; "Fürsorgerinnen in Heeresbetrieben," 116; *BA Koblenz* 12 I/253: Discussion between mining representatives and the DAF Women's Bureau, November 18, 1937. Bethmann, "Betriebswohlfahrtspflege," 177ff, cites the long term factory welfare officer at Knorr-Bremse, Berlin on public health.

109. That this was not an irrelevant point is shown by the fact that 60 percent of the

participants in the mothers' training courses of the Deutsche Frauenwerk were employed, see
Marrenbach, *Fundamente*, 442.
110. Claussen, "Aufgaben," 253.
111. *BA Koblenz*, R 12 I/253: Speech of Scholtz-Klink on May 15, 1936.
112. "The distribution of professions of the husbands of the participants reveals the
following:

	Husbands of the participants in mothers' training courses	Total male working population
Independent	30%	18.8%
Family assistance	—	5.0%
Civil servants	19%	7.9%
Salaried employees	24%	12.7%
Workers	27%	55.6%
	100%	100%

The wives of civil servants, salaried employees, and independents are very heavily
represented: workers' wives, on the other hand, are very poorly represented. Source:
Nachrichtendiest der Reichsfrauenführung, Sonderdienst, vol. 11, no. 2 (February, 1942):
18.

113. "Die Aufgaben der Sozialen Betriebsarbeiterin," *Die Frau* vol. 48, no. 5 (1941):
152.
114. "Vereinbarung zwischen dem Frauenamt der Deutschen Arbeitsfront und dem
Deutschen Frauenwerk," August 20, 1942, in *Nachrichtendiest der Reichsfrauenführung*,
vol. 11, no. 10 (October, 1942): 147f.
115. On the relationship between sexism and racism see: Gisela Bock, "Frauen und ihre
Arbeit im Nationalsozialismus," in *Frauen in der Geschichte*, ed. Annette Kuhn and Gerhard
Schneider (Düsseldorf, 1979), 113–149.
116. Reiche, "Soziale Betriebsarbeiterin," 490.
117. *BA Koblenz*, R 12 I/253: Speech of Scholtz-Klink, May 15, 1936.
118. Traun, "Soziale Betriebsarbeit," 212ff.
119. *BA Koblenz*, R. 12 I/253: Letter from Ganzert to Lohmann November 11, 1936.
120. *Kölnische Zeitung*, no. 232, August 29, 1944, in *BA Koblenz* R 12 I/254.
121. Claussen, "Aufgaben," 253, 252.
122. *BA Koblenz*, R 12 I/253: Speech of Scholtz-Klink, May 15, 1936, and Ganzert to
Lohmann, November 11, 1936.
123. Traun, "Soziale Betriebsarbeit," 212.
124. The files cited here contain several.
125. Nonetheless, individual employers continued to attribute the "increased efficiency
and elevated 'willingness'" of their women workers to the influence of the social workers,
who, after all, were there for that purpose; see Sonnemann, *Landesverteidigung*, 146, 149;
similarly, Traun, "Soziale Betriebsarbeit," 213.
126. Marrenbach, *Fundamente*, 243.
127. "Arbeitswissenschaftliches Institut," "Amt für Berufserziehung und soziale
Betriebsgestaltung" (formerly, DINTA).
128. Traun, "Soziale Betriebsarbeit," 214.
129. Ibid., 214, 211; also "Fürsorgerinnen in Heeresbetrieben," 116.
130. *BA Koblenz*, R 12 I/253: Ganzert to Lohmann, November 11, 1936.
131. *BA Koblenz*, R 12 I/253: DAF brochure "Soziale Arbeit . . ." and discussion
between representatives of mining and the DAF Women's Bureau, November 18, 1937.
132. Reiche, "Soziale Betriebsarbeiterin," 487. "Menschenführung" (leadership) was

also a component of the SIW training courses, see *BA Koblenz*, R 12 I/254: *Programm des Kurses* January 3–14, 1939 and SAA/DAF-SB: Schulungsprogramm vom November 2, 1940.

133. All quotes: BA Koblenz, R 12 I/253: DAF brochure "Soziale Arbeit . . . ".

134. *Kölnische Zeitung*, no. 242, August 24, 1944 in *BA Koblenz*, R 12 I/254.

135. Claussen, "Aufgaben," 262.

136. Scholtz-Klink, *Die Frau im Dritten Reich*, 332ff.; in 1936 Lüders had already recommended factory welfare officers as "technically trained picked troops for the production process," see *Fabrikpflege*, 264.

137. On the National Socialist ideal type of "the German woman" as a doubly dedicated to the "national community" (both as "work comrade" and as "mother of the nation") see Leila Rupp, *Mobilizing Women for War: German and American Propaganda, 1939–1945*, (Princeton, 1978).

138. *BA Koblenz*, R 12 I/263: Eiserhardt to Lohmann, July 17, 1939. Eiserhardt invoked the statements of the social director of IG Farben, Ludwigshafen, Dr. Weiss. Eiserhardt is the author of the unsigned article cited in "Kriegsaufgaben . . . " part I (1939) as well as parts 2 and 3; see also *BA Koblenz*, R 12 I/252: Studders to Trendelenburg, August 31, 1935.

139. "Siemens-Jahresberichte . . . " 1929–30, 1931–32; with a reduced number of employees, the number of cases of support in a year rose 33.5 percent, while cases of financial aid fell by 10 percent (calculated from the data for 1930–31 and 1931–32).

140. Ibid., 1932–33 and 1933–43.

141. Ibid., 1937–38; at this opportunity, financial and material aid could be reduced by 11 percent.

142. See "Kriegsaufgaben . . . " parts 1, 2, and 3; *BA Koblenz*, R 12 I/263: Hilde Eiserhardt to Dr. Reuss (Reichsgruppe Industrie), December 2, 1939.

143. "Siemens-Jahresberichte . . . ," 1938–39.

144. *Jahresberichte der Gewerbeaufsichtsbeamten und Bergbehörden*, issued by the Reich and Prussian Ministry of Labor and Ministry of the Economy, 1933–34, 1935–36, 1937–38 (Berlin, 1935–39).

145. "Kriegsaufgaben . . . ", part I, 303.

146. Ibid., part 2, 326; on lung care, see the "Jahresberichte der Sozialpolitischen Abteilung der Fa. Siemens," SAA 15/Lc 774.

147. "Kriegsaufgaben . . . " part I, 303.

148. Ibid., 304. On monitoring sickness, see also Claussen, "Aufgaben," 252. Family visits were also supposed to prevent facilities being incorrectly "used up." See *Deutsche Arbeitskorrespondenz*, March 17, 1939, "Der Betrieb kümmert sich um die Families" in *BA Koblenz*, 12 I/254.

149. *BA Koblenz*, R 12 I/252: Textile manufacturer Dierig from Langenbielau in Silesia to Reichsgruppe Industrie, October 15, 1935.

150. Hoesch, "Werkpflegeabteilung," 1140.

151. SAA 13/Lc 485 (1925–1952) and many references in the annual reports of the Social Policy Department, SAA 15/Lc 774.

152. "Kriegsaufgaben . . . " part 1, 304; part 2, 326; the example is concerned with the Vereinigten Glanzstoffabriken AG in Kelsterbach.

153. *Nachrichtendienst der Reichsfrauenführung*, vol. 8, no. 4, (April 1939): 159.

154. Preamble to the Law for the Protection of Mothers, May 17, 1942, RGBI. I. 1942, 53, cited from Scholtz-Klink *Die Frau im Dritten Reich*, 339.

155. *Berliner Börsenzeitung*, July 30, 1940, in SAA/DAF-SB.

156. "Siemens-Jahresberichte . . . ," 1937–38 and 1938–39.

157. "Kriegsaufgaben . . . " part 1, 302.

158. Ibid., 303.

159. Ibid., 304.

160. Erich Zängler, "Von der Fürsorge zur Sozialberatung. Die Institution, die man früher Betriebsfürsorge nannte und die jetzt Sozialberatung heisst, wurde vor kurzem 60 Jahre

alt," *Siemens Mitteilungen* 2 (1973): 21–23. At Siemens—at least in one case that I know—a foreign workers' dormitory was supervised by the plant social service worker of the firm that ran it.

161. It must be borne in mind that the records may not be entirely accurate here. If the plant welfare officers' behavior deviated from the official regulations for the treatment of foreign workers ("stern" but "fair" in the context of German racial superiority), it would not have been recorded in the files. This would be the case whether their treatment was distinguished by a greater degree of care and attention, or, on the other hand, by especially "severe standards."

162. *Der Angriff*, June 27, 1940: "'SB-Arbeiterin' unentbehrlich" in SAA/DAF-SB.

163. Claussen, "Aufgaben," 252.

164. *Nachrichtendienst der Reichsfrauenführung* (Sonderdruck, August 1940).

165. "Zum Arbeitseinsatz der Frau in Industrie und Handwerk. Die biologisch bedingten Leistungsvoraussetzungen sowie ihre Beachtung beim Arbeitseinsatz," *Jahrbuch 1940–41*, vol. 1, Arbeitswissenschaftliches Institut der Deutschen Arbeitsfront, (Berlin), 385. Compare Tröger, Frau.

166. Eberhard Pflaume, "Frau und Betrieb," *RKW-Nachrichten*, vol. 14, no. 8 (1940): 97.

167. *BA Koblenz*, R 12 I/336: Special report on work discipline in Gau Bayreuth. I learned of this source from Tilla Siegel.

168. SAA/DAF-SB: Discussion between von Witzleben and Scholtz-Klink, February 26, 1942; "Siemens-Jahresbericht. . . . ," 1942–45. The firm made it clear that "Siemens' industrial welfare system had already been expanded in practice because of the increased use of women during the war, and the firm management had decided to reorganize this work without the influence of the DAF." See SAA/DAF-SB: file note, April 14, 1942.

169. Lüders, "Fabrikpflege," 266.

170. *Nachrichtendienst der Reichsfrauenführung*, vol. 11, no. 3 (March 1942): 33.

171. Claussen, "Aufgaben," 254.

172. SAA/DAF-SB: File note, April 3, 1943. On the refusal of industry to increase half-time work and the attempts to avoid the assignment of conscripted German women by "hoarding" foreign workers, Winkler, *Frauenarbeit*, 138ff.

173. Heinz Boberach, ed. *Meldungen aus dem Reich. Auswahl aus den geheimen Lageberichten des Sicherheitsdienstes der SS 1939–1944* (Berlin, 1965), especially no. 189, May 26, 1941, p. 148–51, and no. 356, February 4, 1943, p. 347–52. See also Winkler. *Frauenarbeit*, 137–42: in her writing one must, however, put up with her use of "aversion to work," (98–100 and passim) which she—in an embarrassing appropriation of the original National Socialist tone—uses to characterize the various forms of refusal to work and the overwork of women, in order to demonstrate a "stubborn passive resistance" to the armaments manufacturers.

174. At Siemens half of all women workers were married by 1942; see SAA 14/Lt 397: Notes on the report made during the visit of Gauleiter Sauckel (Plenipotentiary-General for Labor Allocation), September 25, 1942, 14 ff.

175. In the middle of 1944, when there was hardly enough paper available to carry on their exchange of letters, the Reichsgruppe Industrie was still negotiating about this problem; see *BA Koblenz* R 12 I/254: Protokollniederschrift über eine Sitzung der Reichsgruppe Industrie, May 9, 1944.

176. At the same time there were only 120,000, that is, one tenth as many, kindergarten slots in the U.S. (See Rupp, *Mobilizing*, 171.).

177. Assessor Hermann Willmer, "Der Arbeitseinsatz der verheirateten Frau und seine Wirkung auf die Ehe," *Die Frau*, vol. 48, no. 4 (1941): 115.

178. Ibid., 116.

179. *Nachrichtendienst der Reichsfrauenführung*, vol. 11, no. 9 (September 1942): 123.

180. Letter from the soldier Lange, to the Labor Office in Niesky (Oberlausitz) August

6, 1941, in von Gersdorff, *Kriegsdienst*, 346. These events drew a significant amount of attention from the state authorities, the Party and the armed forces.

181. SAA/DAF-SB: File note from April 3, 1943 on a discussion between industrial social workers of various Berlin firms, DAF Women's leaders, and Labor Office leaders.

182. SAA/14Lt 397: Visit of Sauckel to Siemens (Berlin) September 25, 1942, p. 14.

183. Compare Willmer, "Arbeitseinsatz," 116; Claussen, "Aufgaben," 250; "Kriegsaufgaben . . . ," 1939, part 1: 304 and part 2: 326f.

184. *NS-Frauenwarte*, vol. 11, no. 2 (July 1942): 19.

185. "Kriegsaufgaben . . . ," 1939, part 1: 302.

186. *BA Koblenz*, R 12 I/263: Eiserhardt to Lohmann, July 10, 1939 (concerning the Merck firm, Darmstadt).

187. This setting of goals was explicitly formulated by IG-Farben, see "Kriegsaufgaben . . . ," 1939, part 2: 326 (the author was in close contact with the head of personnel of IG-Farben, Dr. Weiss) as well as at Merck, Darmstadt. See BA Koblenz, R 12 I/263; Eiserhardt to Lohmann July 10, 1939.

188. It should be noted, however, that industrial social work does not provide an appropriate context for analysing the relationship between industrial capitalism in Germany and the National Socialist version of genocidal racism.

189. See Tilla Siegel, "Lohnpolitik im nationalsozialistischen Deutschland," in Carola Sachse, et al., *Angst, Belohnung, Zucht und Ordnung: Herrschaftsmechanismen im Nationalsozialismus* (Opladen, 1982), 59–139.

190. For this see the AWI's study, "Zum Arbeitseinsatz der Frau in Industrie und Handwerk. Die biologisch bedingten Leistungsvoraussetzungen sowie ihre Beachtung beim Arbeiteinsatz," *Jahrbuch 1940–41* vol. 1, Institute of Labor Science of the DAF (Berlin), 373–418; this is exhaustively cited in Tröger, "Frau", 264–60.

191. This is emphasized by Annemarie Tröger in her discussion of the DAF Institute of Labor Science, where she suggests that it adopted as its position on women's work the double burden of the new female proletariat created by the process of rationalization. The Institute's position thus resembled that of employers and was highly realistic in the sense that it proposed as an employment strategy what was actually happening in the factories; see "Frau ."

192. Winkler adopts this position when she believes the absence of the universal obligation must be attributed to Hitler's ideological blindness; see, *Frauenarbeit*, 187–91.

193. Bock, "Frauen", and "Abtreibung und Sterilisation unterm Nationalsozialismus", *Journal für Geschichte* 6 (1980). Gabriele Czarnowski, "Frauen-Staat-Medizin. Aspekte der Körperpolitik im Nationalsozialismus," *Beiträge zur feministischen theorie und praxis* 14 (1985).

194. *BA Koblenz* R 12 I/253: Speech by Scholtz-Klink, May 15, 1936. In this she echoes the eugenic views of the War Office's Center for Women's Labor in the First World War. These were revived and widely publicized in 1936–1939, including by women who had worked for the Center, in order to emphasize the serious consequences of women's work in a future war—the adverse effect on their health and the danger of eugenically-damaging reproductive disorders—and to stress the necessity of preventive measures in the field of eugenics and of family social policy.

Index